Sick & Tired Series

Sick and Tired

Empathy, Encouragement, and

Practical Help for Those

Suffering with Chronic Illness

KIMBERLY RAE

Praise for *Sick and Tired*

As an employee at a Christian bookstore, there are very few books out there touching on this subject. It would be wonderful to have this book in our bookstore. I think it would greatly help those with chronic illnesses, as well as those who might have a friend or relative struggling with one.

> *~ Grawyn Miller, Leap of Faith Christian Bookstore*

The book I've been waiting for has finally been written! I will be referring to this book often—for practical tips, laughter, and sound, biblical advice when the road is feeling long. *Sick and Tired* was the pick-me-up I needed.

> *~ Bethany, MS since 2003*

Loving what I'm reading. I think this book is necessary. I haven't seen any out there like this one.

> *~ Tammy, herniated disc in back since 2008*

I was almost jaded when I first cracked *Sick and Tired* open. What could Kimberly Rae offer me that the medical profession and so many others couldn't? The amount of practical wisdom in *Sick and Tired*, delivered with wit and humor, is well worth a read! I plan to gift this book to several people. Consider this book your prescription for surviving and thriving with health challenges.

> *~ Jen, Raynaud's Phenomenon and food allergies since 2006*

Everybody pretty much in the United States is in some sort of disease state.

> *~ Larry A. Law, Glycobiology instructor*

Dedication

To Brian, with thanks for sticking with me
in sickness and in health
and in sickness
…and sickness
…and sickness.
I love you.

Author Acknowledgments

To every person who believed I was genuinely sick before I got an official diagnosis, thank you. That means more than you can imagine.

For everyone who understands when I have to say no to another activity, when I have to wave off your amazing dessert, and when I have to admit I just can't keep up with you, I thank you.

To my family, who has supported me and been there through so many health crises, loving me in so many different ways—I love you and appreciate you!

Thank you, Brian, for listening to me analyze and critique and go on about hundreds of symptoms and what they could possibly all add up to mean. You must have been drowning in information overload—or boredom—but you still listened, and your solid strength through my crazy upheaval has meant the world to me.

Thank you, Eddie Jones and Lighthouse Publishing, for deciding this message was one the world needs. On behalf of all of us "sickies," we appreciate the recognition that we need encouragement.

Thank you, Andrea Merrell, my very first official editor, for your vote of confidence, and for not telling me to start over.

Thank you, John McPherson, for adding your humor to this project. Your cartoons are my favorite part of the book.

Most importantly, thank you to my Jesus, the One who chose me, broke me, limited me, and held me close. Going through this fire has been awful, but going through it with You has made it bearable. Thanks for showing me that You can do more with my being less than I ever could have done, being what I thought was more.

Table of Contents

Introduction

Be careful about reading health books.
You may die of a misprint.

Mark Twain

Sometimes I want to slap a sticky note on my forehead that says, "I am sick. No, I don't look sick at this moment. But I am not faking having a disease just because I'm not in a wheelchair, and I am not a freak."

Now, I am aware walking around with a note like that on my head would actually put me in the freak category. Not to mention all those words would only fit on a Post-It note if I wrote very, very small, and then people would have to get close to me to read it, and that might just put me over the edge. I'm really into my personal space.

The thing is, I don't like talking about having chronic health problems that interfere with my life. I don't like the way people look down, over, and around me when they realize I have a chronic illness. Or worse yet, the suspicious way their eyes narrow when they decide it's all in my head, or I'm a hypochondriac.

Why does it bother me to tell people I have health problems? Doesn't everybody at some point? I suppose that's the crux right there. For most people, the difference is in the "some point" part. They have a problem. They go to the doctor. Doctor fixes it. Life moves on. It was a small, annoying inconvenience.

For me, and likely for you since you're reading this, your problem is not so temporary. You've got it for life, or until science finds a cure, which for some diseases is as likely as winning the lottery when you haven't ever bought a ticket. So we make people nervous.

Nobody wants to have a condition that affects their social outings, work choices, family life, and just general day-to-day stuff. Nobody picks that for what they want to be when they grow up. "Oh teacher!" The kindergartener excitedly raises his hand. "When I grow up, I want to have a chronic illness and have people say how strong and courageous I am for enduring it even though I don't have any choice in the matter!" Woo-hoo.

Instead, Americans spend billions trying to avoid anything that even smells like sickness. Our country has enough pills, vitamins, and herbal remedies to make you sick even if you started out healthy, or at least to make your urine turn neon yellow—which is an interesting phenomenon but likely not worth all the money it took to make it happen.

We all desperately want to be well. And why not? Being well means you get to be as active as you want to be and in charge of your own daily schedule: How much sleep to get. What to eat. What job to choose, or how many children to have.

For those of us with chronic illness, we've had to give up some or all of those freedoms. And they probably didn't seem like freedoms at the time. We likely took them for granted until our bodies took them from us. Now here we are, active brains inside limited, broken bodies. But as technology has yet to create a way to get an entire body transplant, we're stuck with it.

Unless, of course, you have a neurological problem, as I think I might, in which case I'm sorry about your brain. Getting a brain transplant is a seriously bad idea. You would not even know who you were, and would not appreciate how much better you were feeling.

I would like to trade in my health problems and be well again. I sometimes think that would be getting my life back. But the truth is, this is my life, and as I have come to (almost) accept that fact and make the best of it, I think there's hope for me.

Maybe not to cease being a freak to some, but to cease seeing myself as a victim, as a traumatic case, or even as a lesser being because of my illness.

That being the goal, maybe I'll remove the hypothetical Post-It note from my forehead and put it in my back pocket, to be removed periodically and waved in people's faces only when I'm having a tough day.

It's a start anyway.

Chapter One

Joining the Club—Involuntarily

Go away. I'm all right.
Last Words of H. G. Wells

I suppose I should tell you how I ended up in this unhealthy club, considering you're reading this book and I wrote it and all. Apparently my problems started in childhood, just little things here and there that seemed odd, but nothing major enough to be concerned about. By high school I knew I was different. I didn't play sports, and that whole running a mile in P.E. was awful. I figured I was a wimp and if I could ever just garner up some gumption I'd be able to keep up.

Every winter for as long as I could remember, I'd catch a nasty cold, take lots of meds that left me feeling like a zombie, and sleep, sleep, sleep. I actually kind of looked forward to the two weeks of resting and not expecting anything from myself. You'd think that would have been a clue, but hey, it was my normal, so how was I to know I was weird?

In college I was so, so tired. (I know you're nodding your head on that one!) For my two required P.E. classes I chose ice skating and sailing—the two I figured wouldn't make me run a mile. Halfway through college I got a bad bout of bronchitis. I jumped back into classes and regular life before I should have because I felt guilty for still needing to recover past what seemed a normal time. I didn't want to look lazy or people thinking I was making excuses.

It was around that time my mother noticed I could go from being excited and happy to stressed and (blush) crabby within minutes. With a history of diabetes in our family, she mentioned I needed to get my blood sugar tested.

And here began my strange experiences with extremely interesting doctors. The doctor I went to told me to go to McDonald's and eat a breakfast high in sugar, then come back and he would check my blood. That sounded fun, so I obeyed. He checked my sugar and told me, yep, I had hypoglycemia. He gave me a paper on what foods I could and couldn't eat and that was the end of it.

My whole world shifted. I was supposed to do a major overhaul in my daily schedule and my meal choices—everything I would or would not put in my mouth.

This was a big deal. Why was I the only one who thought so?

Well, since nobody was going to throw me a hey-your-life-just-got-wacked-with-a-chronic-issue party, I did the changes myself, though not very well. Back then I wasn't into doing my own research, and that sheet of paper the doctor gave me didn't exactly guide me like the Star of Bethlehem.

Right before my senior year of college, I got what I assumed was a stomach flu. I got lots of *supposed* stomach flu-like symptoms, as if stomach bugs just followed me around like a bunch of groupies. I threw up so many times and so violently, blood vessels all over my eyeballs burst. What a great way to show up senior year. Friends would see me from a distance and say, "Hey, Kim! How was your—what happened to *you*?" I looked like ... well, I don't know. I'd never seen anything like it. I had red polka-dots all over my eyeballs, like they had measles. I didn't get asked out on any dates during those weeks.

Anyway, after college I went to Bangladesh for two years. Great idea for someone with health problems, right? Well, I just thought I had low blood sugar and it was manageable enough. I taught a little in a school and loved the chaos and color of living in one of the most crowded places in the world.

I could write about that for pages, but suffice it to say that after a few years and several strange health "events," it was clear I had problems beyond hypoglycemia.

The biggest problem, however, was nobody could figure out what my problem was. I went to a whole plethora of doctors and got tested for just about everything imaginable. (I'm feeling your empathy as you read this. Thanks.) And each time I'd get my hopes up thinking maybe this time they'd find this elusive problem I had and it would get fixed.

Then the doctor would walk in, smile benignly, and tell me my blood tests came back normal.

"Isn't that good?"

"NO!" I wanted to shout.

I'd leave yet another doctor's office with my fifty-three symptoms, but no diagnosis.

Between then and now, I've had so many needles in my veins, they've rolled and collapsed and I had to have a Central IV put in. I've watched nurses put on face masks because they thought I had the bird flu. I had pneumonia and pleurisy and bacteremia, but I'd lived in Indonesia so they kind of freaked out and put me in the mental room—okay, so it was because they didn't have any other available ER rooms, but it still felt rather personal. I've had doctors tell me I was their most complicated case—always encouraging to hear—and got a three hundred and ninety-five dollar consultation bill from an expert who told me to "eat right and exercise more."

I've had pre-eclampsia, eclampsia, and seizures. After the seizures there are two whole days I don't remember when people came to visit me in the hospital. Hopefully, I was nice to them. I've had fluid on my brain and three major doctors gathered in my hospital room trying to decide which of the two life-threatening treatments to try. I've been lectured for letting my potassium get critically low. Who knew you could have a heart attack from low potassium? Not me, but I do now. Every once in a while I've been happy to have a sugar low because it meant I got to eat something fun.

Also, along the way, I've met some of the nicest, most kind and considerate doctors and nurses on the planet, and given thanks for good medical care. After living in the third world, you really learn to be thankful for things like sanitation and not having to bring your own bedding with you to the hospital.

And now, just this past year, after fifteen years of searching, scores and scores of hours of personal research on the computer, and ridiculous attempts at diets and treatments trying to fix something, I have been officially diagnosed. Seems it wasn't all in my head after all.

It's in my adrenals. A homeopathic doctor told me that very thing years ago after a saliva test, but ever since then, because it wasn't an "official" diagnoses, I couldn't get any "real" doctors to take it seriously. I'd have to go off the medication to do testing, which I did once for seven weeks of major misery, to be told, once again, the test results came back fine and I didn't need to be on the medicine at all. They couldn't tell me why I was unable to function without it, just that I didn't need it.

Now, after all that, I have been diagnosed by a pituitary specialist at Emory. I have Addison's disease. I also have asthma—which happened somewhere in the middle of all this and was quite annoying as I really didn't have time for another condition—and of course, the low blood sugar thing, and scoliosis, which means my spine has a nice pretty curve in a place where it shouldn't. My most recent addition has been finding a cyst in the middle of my head. Now this did strike me as funny because, technically, if it's been causing a lot of my problems, then it's safe to say it really was in my head all this time after all.

All that to say ... I do have a chronic health condition, and thus am qualified to write this book. Now, let's move on to your story, and how to explain your condition to people who don't want to read a big, long chapter like the one I just wrote.

If you didn't want to read it, sorry, but it's kind of too late now.

Individual Or Group Study Questions

1. Think back. How long have you been suffering with symptoms?

2. When did you first approach a doctor with your symptoms? Did he take them seriously?

3. What are your feelings right now about having chronic health problems?

4. Do you have a diagnosis yet? Do you feel it is complete and covers your entire illness?

ACTIVITY: Consider journaling your entire health story, starting from whenever you first experienced symptoms until now. It's a good way to consolidate years of information and emotions into one place and will give you a reference point for future use. Also, you'll have the whole story to hand over to whoever wants to know about it on those days you don't feel like telling it.

CLOSE TO HOME JOHN McPHERSON

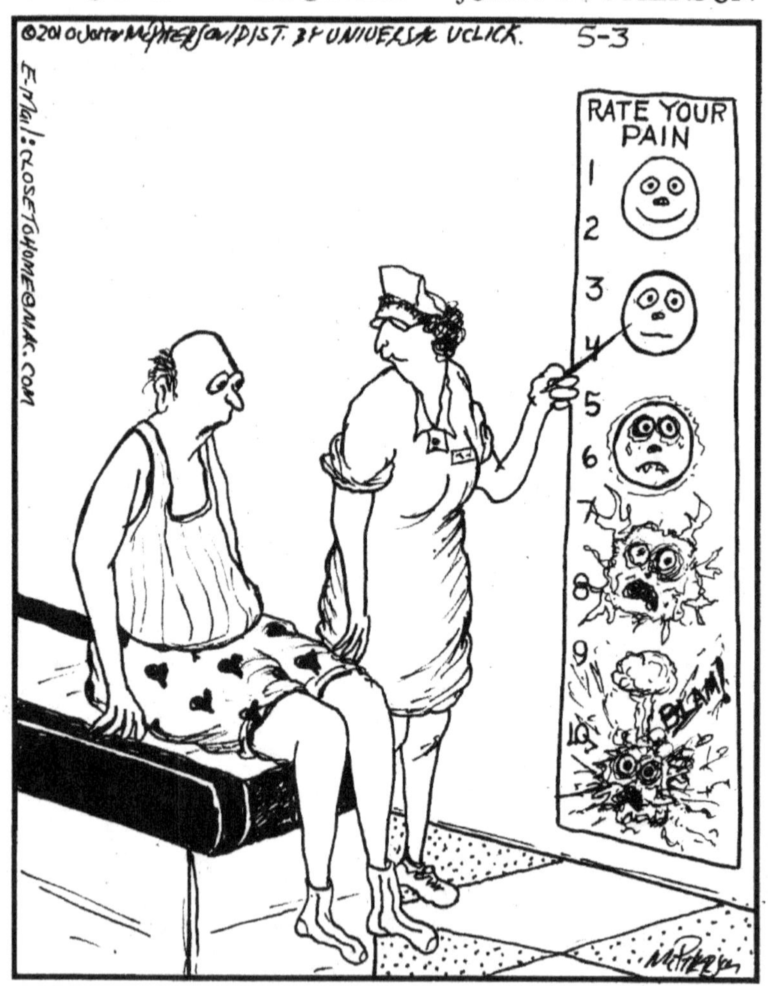

Chapter Two

So What's Your Problem?

Quit worrying about your health. It'll go away.
Robert Orben

Most of the time when people ask me about my condition, I don't have time to rattle off fifteen years of health misadventures. Their eyes would likely roll back in their heads trying to process everything in one earful anyway. It was kind of fun telling you in that last chapter, though, because you know there is so much more to the story: finding something that might define the problem, chasing it down, getting hopes up, being disappointed, giving up, then finding something else and starting the process all over again.

For the general public, however, that long process is horrifying—not that it's not to us, but we're stuck with it—and they would prefer a simplified, more concise version of the long, long story. Kind of like saying, "The pilgrims sailed to America," or "The Civil War was bad."

So what's your story? When someone asks you about your health condition, you, like me, likely start picturing years full of scenes and feelings and information. The person watches your eyes glaze over as you try to decide what, out of the hundreds of thoughts, you should actually share. There's so much to say, oftentimes we end up standing there with our mouths open, not actually saying anything because our brains get clogged up with information and it's all too mashed together for any one sentence to actually make it out.

This, unfortunately, gives the impression that maybe we really are making this up, since we can't even give an answer about what our problem is. Therefore, let's think through how to fix this dilemma. The following little section will help you bring things down to a concise, simplified format to give people enough information for their initial generic health question. If they want to know more, they can ask.

This is particularly important for those of you who tend to avoid any reference to, or outward showing of, having a health problem at all, because you don't want people to think you're complaining, blaming God, or whatever.

First things first. When people find out you have a health problem, they ask what it is. Maybe they ask out of curiosity, maybe they want to help, or maybe they think you really don't have a legitimate problem, though this last one is much less likely than we assume it is.

Rather than starting on a long story about how doctors can't figure out what's wrong with you and you were tested for this and that but the results came back fine, and ... and ... and (the person at this point is trying to follow you but probably got lost somewhere back when you were getting tested), we need to communicate in such a way that people leave the conversation knowing we have a health condition, we have limitations, and perhaps even what the largest of those limitations happens to be.

To do that, we need to start with the big initial question. So, if you don't mind me asking, what is your health problem?

"Well...big long story...not sure...doctors can't find..."

This is not a good answer. I know because I've done it many times, and I go away feeling frustrated and defensive. I have no idea how the other person feels, but I know I don't feel good about my answer.

Here's a better option: "I have a condition that affects my joints. I struggle with a lot of pain so I try to avoid stairs."

If you told me that, I might nod in sympathy. Then I would likely ask another question, since I recognize you do have a legitimate issue because you communicated it confidently to me. I'd feel comfortable asking, since I can tell you aren't upset talking about it, and I would like to know more because learning more about your condition will help me learn more about you.

Give it a try. Say I ask you, "I heard you have a chronic health problem. What is it?"

You pick which option you like best and fill in the blanks.

"I have a disease called _______________________. That means my ___________ doesn't work right, so I have to ___________________."

"I have a condition that affects my _______________. This causes me problems with my _______________ and I can't _________________ anymore."

Saying either of the above does not leave room for people to question whether or not you have a condition. It does leave room, however, for them to ask you more about it, which is a good thing. From there, you can move on to comments such as the following:

"I struggle with having to give up _________________. I've had this condition for ____________, so I've learned to ______________________."

"I really miss being able to _______________________, but I've learned to ask for help with _________________, and that has been a blessing because _______________."

I find if I can end the comment positively, people know I'm not feeling devastated about my condition (at least not at that moment) and they can ask me deeper questions, giving me a chance to honor God as well as express my limitations in a setting that doesn't make me feel inferior or guilty.

You may find that just learning to express your condition in one concise sentence, calmly and with confidence, makes you feel much less like a victim of sickness and more like a person who happens to be sick. Defining it keeps it from defining you.

Having said all that, rather than the entire last chapter you just waded through, here's my answer in a nutshell:

"Hi, my name is Kim. I have Addison's disease. That means my adrenal glands don't work like they should, so I'll have to take steroids every day for the rest of my life. I wear out easily and have to rest sometimes when I don't want to, which is why I'm going to sit down now. Would you like to join me?"

Individual Or Group Study Questions

1. Do you feel overwhelmed when people ask you about your condition?

2. Do you catch yourself telling them a long story that leaves you frustrated and them confused?

3. Do you feel like people don't take your condition seriously because it isn't diagnosed yet, or is an "invisible" illness like fibromyalgia or chronic fatigue?

4. Do you ever think people are picking up on your own insecurities about your illness?

5. If you could communicate with confidence, do you think that would change how people respond?

ACTIVITY: Fill in the blanks in the sentences in this chapter, then type and print the sentences that express you best. Put them on a 3x5 card and carry them around until you memorize exactly how you want to present your illness to others.

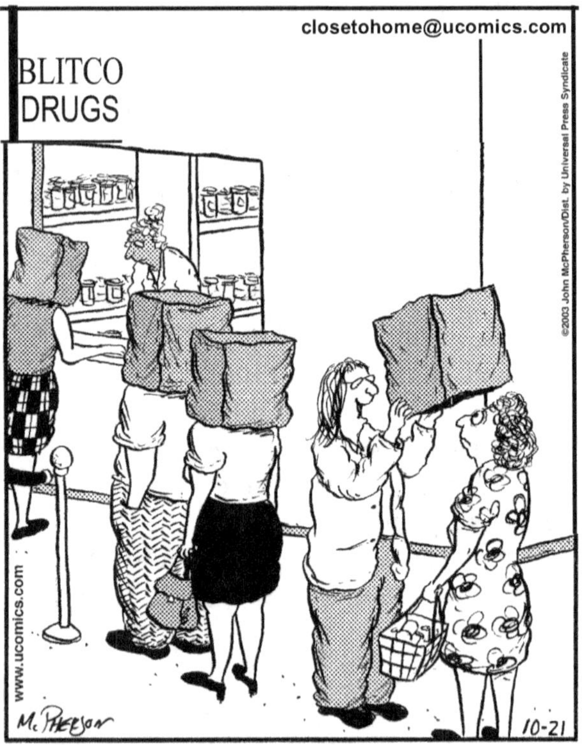

"It's part of the government's new emphasis on patient privacy, ma'am."

Chapter Three

Sit Down and Cry About It

Sometimes a scream is better than a thesis.

Ralph Waldo Emerson

You're sitting high up on that examination table with way more of your body exposed than is reasonable, cold air wafting through the cracks in the paper towel they call a gown, your legs dangling like a toddler's, and your heart racing because ... well, because anybody in a setting that makes them feel like a naked toddler is going to feel slightly traumatized. You're desperately hoping for good news while trying to mentally prepare yourself for the worst.

The doctor enters the scene, a nice enough person, but unaware of your trauma and seemingly unaffected by the fact that you're looking at him like he holds your future in his hands. He doesn't, not really, but his knowledge of your body and its ability, or lack thereof, to function will determine a large chunk of your life from this moment on.

He looks at you and gives some word, usually a nice long one that sounds very official. "You have

________________________________." He may give a little more information, or a brochure. Or maybe he'll pat you on the shoulder like one doctor did to me, and give you a whole handful of papers on depression. *Thanks, Doctor ... suddenly I'm feeling depressed.*

And now, despite all your hopes and plans and goals for your life, you are part of a large group of people *defined* and *confined* by chronic illness—a very large group. The Center for Disease Control posted that 133 million Americans—nearly one out of every two people—had at least one chronic illness. The Census Bureau projected that 96% of those illnesses are invisible, suffered by people who "may look perfectly healthy."

It's not a place any of us would like to be. In fact, many of us have worked very hard and searched very long for a solution, some treatment or exercise or surgery or information that would get us out of this group and back to "normal."

There is a real and legitimate feeling of grief that hits when we first encounter this new, unhappy reality. When you first find out, or when things digress, you need to allow yourself to go through the process of loss, including the natural feelings of anger, disbelief, helplessness, and fear. Don't pretend those away by trying to be spiritual or strong. Give yourself some time to grieve, with the knowledge that you must not choose to set up camp there. In time, you'll need to get up and move forward.

What's a good time frame for grieving? I can't give you a number; that's something between you and God. I know for me, I can deal with a difficult crisis like surgery pretty quickly, but when I found out I had an incurable disease and just had to live with it, the news hit me hard. I found myself emotionally eating and not wanting to talk with people on the phone for a few days. I felt guilty, knowing they wanted to hear the news and encourage me, but I wasn't ready to hear how God had a reason for this and it would work out for good, etc. I knew all those things were true, but I needed to grieve first.

I asked my husband to answer the phone and update people, and to admit to them I was struggling. I allowed myself to be encouraged through their acts of love and cards instead of pretending I was fine like I was tempted to do. Going through all of that helped. Now I feel much more able to face this new reality and adapt to it, because I faced and accepted what was lost.

I'm no expert on loss and how to deal with it, but my guess would be that most of us are going to go through variations of four categories:

1. **Stunned**—overwhelmed, feeling this can't be really happening to us.

2. **Emotional**—anger, denial, tears, depression, and a whole host of feelings in response to the fact we don't like this and want out.

3. **Broken**—recognizing our helplessness and inability to deal with this or conquer it.

4. **Accepting**—coming to grips with God's plan even if we don't understand it, and letting God put His strength in place of our weakness.

When Job lost *everything*, and I mean everything, the first thing he did was go through the rituals of grieving common at that time—shaved his head, tore his clothes—then he *fell down and worshipped* (Job 1:20). He verbally recognized God had the right to give and take away.

Afterward, he didn't bounce back up and pretend nothing had happened. The Bible says Job's friends came over and were so overwhelmed about what happened to him they all sat in silence for seven days, which was a wise thing to do. It was only when they started opening their mouths to offer advice their helpfulness went down the drain.

I think this fits under the stunned category. We hear the news we've got a condition with no cure, or we have no diagnosis yet but it's become clear our symptoms are not going to go away. We walk around in a fog, not able to really process the facts. It's as if we have a new file labeled "illness" and we can't figure out where to put it in our mental file box. There's no room in the file box for this particular file. How did this happen?

Once Job's friends started talking—blaming him for what happened, saying he must have done something wrong—Job moved into the next category and got emotional. If you read the book of Job in the Bible, you hear him verbalizing the injustice of what happened to him. He complains about how lousy he feels. He defends his own righteousness. He even wishes he had never been born.

For some reason, his friends don't do much listening, except to come up with ammunition for their next comments. They keep pushing their own opinions down poor Job's throat until Job hits the third category—completely broken, without hope, without anything. Even his wife tells him to curse God and die. No more arguments, only a powerlessness in the face of a reality which cannot be changed.

This is the point where God steps in. When we are in the emotional part, God understands and holds us in our pain. When, however, we hit the stage of brokenness, where the feelings haven't fixed the problem and we recognize this isn't going away no matter how we fight or rant or hate it, it's as if the feelings drain away, leaving a deep dark hole headed toward despair.

In this place, however, if we are willing, God can come through. For Job, God entered the scene and reminded him of some very important truths, basically all making the point that God is God, He has the right to do whatever He wants, and even though we don't understand His ways, we need to humble ourselves before Him regardless.

This may seem unfair. God never did tell Job why he had to go through all that horror. We know from the Biblical account that eternal questions were being answered by whether Job was faithful or not. It was a really big deal, way bigger than Job ever could have imagined. However, once Job saw God for who He really was, he fell to the ground and recognized his own humanity in the face of God's deity. It was after, when Job prayed for his friends (acceptance, despite what others thought or did), God blessed Job and changed his life for the better.

None of us want to be a Job. We know the story has helped millions through the ages find comfort and help, but we still would rather it be someone else's story rather than our own.

For some unfathomable reason, however, God has chosen us. Not because we volunteered, not because we *want* our faithfulness through suffering to help others, but because God has some unseen, eternally important reason we cannot, at present, comprehend.

Knowing this, we can fall down and worship, give ourselves time to go through the feelings of anger or despair, but then come out stronger on the other end. Not because we ourselves have strength, but because we have accepted God's will, and in doing so can receive the strength He offers.

So give yourself time and room to grieve. Don't stuff all the feelings away, pretending they aren't there. Talk to someone about how you feel. Journal your thoughts or simply cry out to God. He can handle it; just read some of the stuff David said in the Psalms, and God called him a man after His own heart. In time, after you are exhausted emotionally and have no more strength to fight, you can choose to move on to acceptance, and from there ... well, that's for the next chapter.

P.S. Grief is not a one-time thing for people with chronic health problems. Just like people grieving the loss of a loved one find the sadness washes over them at holidays or family events or even unexpected everyday moments, we who are grieving the loss of ourselves, or our former lives, will find the feelings come at random—when someone mentions an activity we used to love, or even something as simple as bumping against a door frame, or not being able to find our keys. It doesn't mean you're a failure. It means you're human. And it's okay.

Then Job arose, tore his robe, and shaved his head; and he fell to the ground and worshiped. And he said: "Naked I came from my mother's womb, and naked shall I return there. The LORD gave, and the LORD has taken away; blessed be the name of the LORD." In all this Job did not sin nor charge God with wrong. Job 1:20-22

<u>Individual Or Group Study Questions</u>

1. Have you ever thought about the fact that having a chronic illness involves genuine loss and deserves to be grieved?

2. How did you feel immediately after hearing you had a condition, or when you realized your symptoms were not going to go away?

3. Right now, do you think you are in the Stunned, Emotional, Broken, or Accepting category?

4. Where do you feel like you should be at this point?

5. What do you think a reasonable time for grieving should be for you personally?

6. Do you think brokenness is necessary before acceptance, or can that part be skipped? Why or why not?

ACTIVITY: Give yourself permission to grieve. What would best help you go through this process? Some ideas would be journaling, praying, talking with a trusted friend or counselor, or getting away for a couple of days.

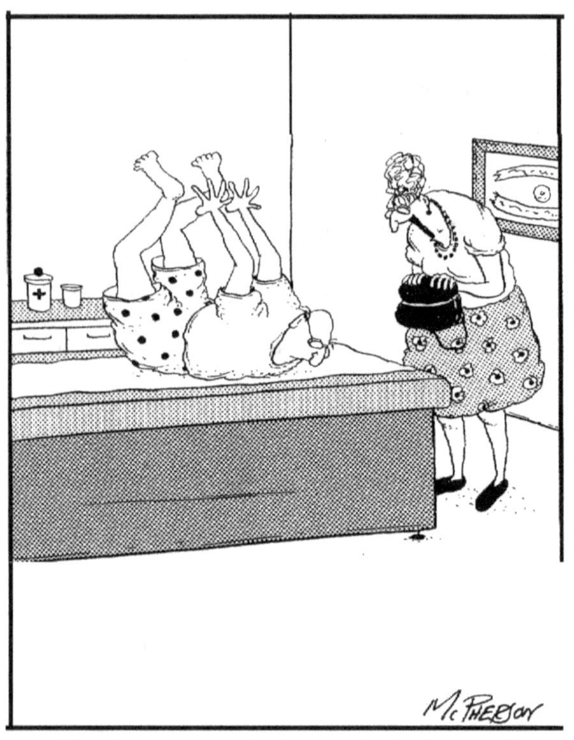

'The doctor says it's just a pinched nerve."

Chapter Four

It's Not Fair

*My doctor recently told me that jogging could add years to my life.
I think he was right. I feel ten years older already.*

Milton Berle

I grew up in a military family. Whenever the Navy decided to transfer my dad to another post, they didn't call him up and ask if he felt personally inclined to pack up his family and move. No one asked us kids if we felt like leaving our friends and becoming the new kids at some other school. They assigned a new spot; we moved.

How we dealt with it, however, was our own choice.

People throughout history have found themselves in new, unwanted settings, and have had to decide how they would choose to react. Think of the women on the wagon train who left nice amenities and friends and family in the East to go wandering out west, riding a rickety wagon for months—MONTHS (makes my rear hurt just thinking about it). And then, if they actually made it, they had to adapt to a whole new climate and culture, maybe not having any neighbors for miles, which would be a big deal if you had to walk over there every time you needed to borrow some butter or sugar.

If you read *Little House on the Prairie*, you get this overall happy, cozy feeling about such things, but only because Laura Ingalls Wilder chose to see life that way. Others in the same situation got cabin fever, went into deep depression, went insane, or worse.

Same situation, different responses.

So let's talk about you. You've been "transferred" from your former easier life to this new, more difficult one. You didn't pick this transfer; it was chosen for you.

The question is, how will you deal with it?

When I, a southerner, married my husband, who is from Ohio, my first winter in Ohio was not fun. I was used to Florida, Georgia, and tropical countries like Indonesia. I had no experience with snow that actually stayed on the ground for hours...days...weeks...forever it seemed.

That first winter was hard. Initially I just wouldn't accept the fact of a long winter. I complained and felt like Ohio was against me (amazing how egocentric we get when we don't feel well). I finally decided to stop hiding from the winter, but when I'd get out in it, I would still only do my usual southern version of keeping warm and end up getting sick, again thinking Ohio was somehow elongating this winter thing on purpose just to make me miserable. At long last, I learned from those who lived there about a wonderful thing called layering. I learned to put on several layers of clothing, adding scarves, mittens and a hat to my normal open-coat routine.

With a few changes in habit, Ohio turned out to be not such a bad place after all. I still didn't enjoy the fact of the long winter, but I was able to enjoy life within it.

The way I see it, anyone unfortunately ushered into the world of chronic health problems has three choices:

1. **Refuse to Accept It**—run away from the reality in protest, hide from people, complain, get bitter. Result: you and everyone around you becomes miserable, and it still doesn't make the problem go away.

2. **Accept but Don't Adapt**—decide to live with this new condition, but don't change any habits. Result: you end up even more unhealthy, you begin to feel like a victim and see yourself as helpless, and you and concerned loved ones are still miserable, but more of a *confused* miserable as opposed to an angry miserable.

3. **Accept and Adapt**—recognize this is your new world and try to learn how to live well within it. You change things—some big, some small—to make the everyday struggles easier. Result: you likely will never love having a health condition, but you will learn to live with joy within the condition.

None of us chose to have a chronic health condition, but the truth is, this is where we live now, and how we choose to feel, think, and act will matter not only to our own future but also the future of those we love.

Individual Or Group Study Questions

1. Do you believe your attitude is your own choice? Why or why not?

2. What would you say your attitude was when you first started having problems?

3. How would you say it is now?

4. Do you know someone who has chosen to become bitter about life's disappointments? How do you feel being around that person? Does this attitude make anything better for the person or their loved ones?

5. Did you go through a stage where you accepted your condition but didn't adapt? Are you in that stage now? Do you see how this is good, but not good enough?

6. How do you get from just accepting to accepting and adapting?

ACTIVITY: Find someone you trust and tell them about the three choices. If you are willing to hear the truth, ask that person where they see you right now. You may learn some things to help you move forward, or be reassured you are on the right track.

CLOSE TO HOME — JOHN MCPHERSON

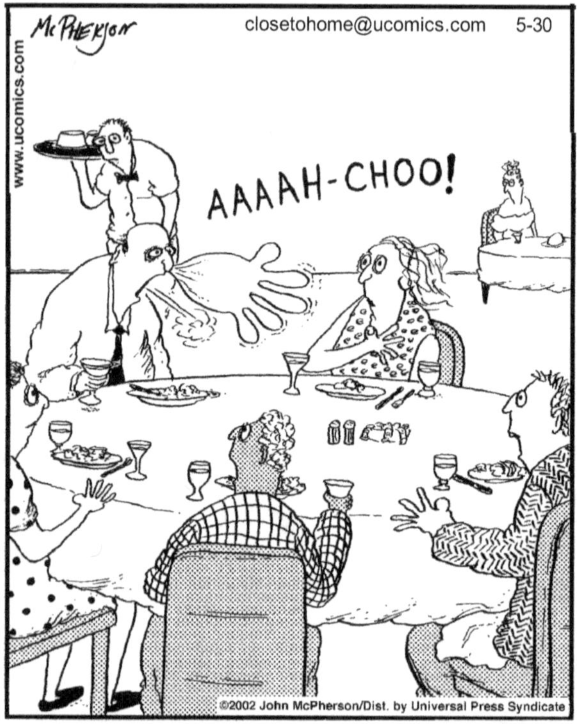

While entertaining some clients, the surgical glove lost inside Tom during his bypass surgery makes an untimely reappearance.

Chapter Five

Running the Yellow Light

What's the two things they tell you are healthiest to eat?
Chicken and fish ...
You know what you should do?
Combine them ... eat a penguin.

Dave Attell

A physical symptom is like a yellow light. You're driving along the road, hitting all green lights along the way, enjoying your favorite music on the radio or chatting with friends. Then suddenly up ahead, the cheerful green turns to a bright yellow hue. You weren't expecting that. You don't like that.

The yellow light is there for a reason. No matter how much you might not want that color to appear, the yellow light is there to tell you a red light is coming. It's a warning sign.

At this point you have two options. You could slow down to a stop, waiting until the light turns back to green, allowing you to continue on as before. Or, and this is probably the first option most of us think of, you can speed up, hoping to run through it before it turns red so you can continue on unhindered. You might even get a rush out of beating the system by making it just in time.

Problem is, if you decide to ignore the warning and speed through the intersection, the light might turn red before you expect and you might find yourself blindsided. You could wake up a few days later to be told your vehicle is in jagged pieces, your body is not much better, and now you have major negative ramifications to deal with because you decided to take the risk.

I'm not here to lecture anybody on taking that risk. Many people in general, and especially Americans, don't like admitting the need to slow down. Slow down? Isn't that just admitting an inner compulsion toward laziness? Isn't it just an excuse? Oh no, we want to keep going, to conquer and come out on top, to say we overcame by our own will or pulling ourselves up by our own bootstraps. Our culture tends to value those who disregard their own bodies' needs to succeed.

I can't tell you the number of times I've chosen to "push through," to keep going and hope my symptoms somehow fixed themselves, or I've mentally argued with myself, trying to decide if I'm making it up, trying to get attention, or jumping the gun before things really needed to be dealt with.

Sometimes I've been able to run the yellow light without any negative results. But we all know that people who run yellow lights on a regular basis are much more likely to end up in a bad accident someday, or several. It took several "bad accidents," health-wise, for me to learn to stop hoping the light would not turn red before I got to the other side.

I am now at the point where, when I see a yellow light, not only do I slow down, but sometimes I even pull over to the side of the road—symptomatically speaking—so I can make sure the brakes work before I get to the intersection.

Okay, so I'm not there all the time yet. In fact, the reason I have time to type all this is because I pushed through a stomach flu and didn't go up on my adrenal meds because I was trying to cut down on them. This ended with me in an urgent care facility getting a shot with a stress dose of hydrocortisone in it. That, plus a round of prednisone, had my daily steroid dose up to six times the amount I had been trying to wean off of. So much for hoping it would fix itself.

I am now up far too late because of the prednisone I had to take right before bed. I suppose I should count my blessings and be thankful my brain is running at ridiculously high speeds, thus helping me get this whole project started at a sprint, but the truth is, I'd rather be sleeping. And it could very well be that none of what I'm saying will make any rational sense to anyone who is not on prednisone, in which case this whole staying up experience will be wasted on the general public.

Back to the yellow lights. My point is, our bodies were made with a phenomenal amount of intricate and amazing functions, and when one or several of those functions stops working as they should, the body very resourcefully gives us a message. The message is usually in the form of something unpleasant, like pain, to let us know something needs to change. Something is wrong. If we ignore these warning signs, the body will send more and more signals, more and more pain, until something important shuts down and we have big-time problems.

Pain is considered a bad thing. Usually when we feel pain, rather than assessing the reason for it, we want to pop a pill or do something to make it go away. I know I do. I don't much care for what it's trying to tell me. I just want it to shut up.

I read a great book once called *Pain, the Gift that Nobody Wants*, about a man who worked with lepers. Lepers don't lose limbs and such because of leprosy. They lose them because leprosy deadens the nerves that cause pain, thus leaving the leper with no signal something is wrong (say a cut on the foot), thus giving them no yellow light, no warning that a problem is coming (infection, gangrene), thus running them right into the intersection, headed for a crash (amputation).

In the end, we should be thankful for the yellow lights. Life would be pretty stressful if lights went straight from green to red. We'd all be slamming on our brakes in a panic, and many more accidents would occur.

In the same way, symptoms should be respected. They are trying to help us effectively respond to what our bodies need at the moment. Don't ignore them. Don't hope they will go away on their own. Just slow down and stop if need be, so you can assess or deal with the problem. Then you can move on down the road with peace of mind, with your car and yourself still in one piece.

<u>Individual Or Group Study Questions</u>

1. Are you a risk taker by nature, or more cautious?

2. When you feel symptoms, which way is closest to your natural reaction?

   - Ignore them and they'll go away.
   - Anger this is happening and refusing to respond to the symptoms.
   - Panic that a serious and dangerous problem is coming.
   - Pop a pill and move on.
   - Jump on the internet and do research, or call your doctor.
   - Medicine fixes everything—give me more.

3. Do you think symptoms are a good thing? What might happen if we didn't have any?

   ACTIVITY: Start a record of your different symptoms. A calendar is a good way to record how you're feeling and when. Mark how you dealt with them and the result. Then the next time they happen, you can go back and check what worked and what didn't.

CLOSE TO HOME JOHN MCPHERSON

closetohome@ucomics.com

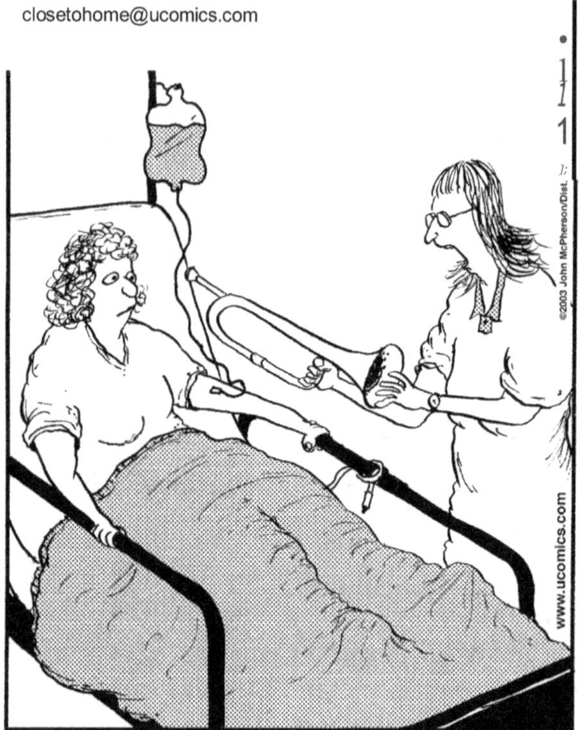

"Here, take this. Our call buttons are broken."

Chapter Six

Choosing the Right Doctor

*Some people think that doctors and nurses
can put scrambled eggs back in the shell.*

Cass Canfield[1]

Some people collect dolls or trains or spoons or model airplanes. I collect doctors.

My collection is rather varied. One doctor's office gave me a beautiful red rose on my first visit. He was a woman's hormone doctor. The man was brilliant. He was the one who said I should never go back overseas considering my condition, and he was surprised I hadn't "kicked off" already. I guess that phrase came out in one of his less-sensitive moments, or maybe he decided I wasn't too hormonal so he could talk like a guy around me.

Another doctor was super nice and I enjoyed visiting him because he was so empathetic, and he enjoyed research, so we'd get together and talk about our latest findings and theories. He'd say I was one of his most complicated cases, which made me feel badly for the permanent worried eyebrow look he had. He never did figure out my problem, but I always felt better after visiting him, so that was something.

Then there was doctor McCracky, or "McQuacky" as my husband not-so-affectionately called him. He had this miniature battering ram that he'd use to whack me on the side of my skull. Did wonders for my hip and back pain for a time, but the treatment was costly and his office far from home. I mentioned once the easier and cheaper option of someone just hitting me over the head with a frying pan, but he – being the serious type – started explaining why that was not a good idea. I kept going, until he decided to ask me questions and check some muscle deep in my hand for the answers. Supposedly my subconscious knew all the answers regarding my health and would tense or not tense that muscle in response. He decided to demonstrate this flakey idea the day I'd convinced a close friend to come visit him to see if he could help her. She never came back, and after that day, neither did I!

You could say that visiting new doctors was a hobby for me—kind of like casual dating. I'd go see a new one, thinking maybe this guy will not only be understanding and easy to talk to, but he'll be a genius and somehow figure out the string of problems I've had all these years.

As you can imagine, most of the time the experience was as disappointing as, well, most casual dates. Maybe not horrible, but not what you're looking for.

Like the older gentleman I went to see who, when I asked why my blood sugar always got messed up the day my period started, gave me that you're-cute-but-female-and-therefore-not-to-be-taken-seriously look (or maybe I was imagining things and he was really thinking about lunch) and said, "Everything gets worse on your period," and he had no idea why it would affect my blood sugar. When I got home, I got online, and wouldn't you know it, there was an answer after all.

One of my chiropractors, Jen, is wonderful. She's a great balance between traditional medicine and holistic. At my last visit, when I showed her my strange muscle bulge with accompanying burn-type mark that's happened several times now (and multiple doctors cannot explain), she talked with me over some possibilities and asked a bunch of questions, then said, "I could speculate on it all day, but I really don't know." She felt badly, but I appreciated her ability to say that so much, I didn't mind. She's told me, "I think doctors get upset when they don't know because we really do want to help." She also says that it bugs her when doctors don't know and they either put the blame on the patient, or call it fibromyalgia. I'm with you, Jen!

My internal doctor in North Carolina was great. She wore cowboy boots and long, flowy skirts. She still had her Wisconsin accent, and one day she actually got out her computer and searched my condition to help answer a question I had. At the time, I wanted to tell her I could do that myself and save us both some time, but it was nice feeling like we were a team.

Which leads me to my point—yes, there is a point here. Doctors are just people. A few of them have helped save my life. A few have made it worse. Can you imagine how tough it must be to see twenty or thirty people in a day, many of them with a weird mixture of symptoms that could be pointing toward any of a score of illnesses, and in twenty minutes you're supposed to figure out what to do next, knowing that person just put their body and their immediate future into your care? Yikes. I wouldn't want to do that. And I'd feel pretty relieved when someone came in with a simple cold. I would be tempted to be overwhelmed when someone came in with fifty-two symptoms (like me), a pile of unusual test results that didn't point to anything specific (like me), and who had been going to doctor after doctor for fifteen years looking for the one who could solve their problem (like me).

I've gotten to where I start apologizing from the get-go!

Over the years, I have learned a bit about the kind of doctor I need. Just like looking for the right guy to date, those of us with chronic issues need to look for the right kind of doctor to work with. Here are some of the qualities necessary for a good chronic-illness doctor:

1.   **One who doesn't make you feel you're a burden.** Who wants to go visit a doctor who makes you feel guilty merely for being there? We don't need any more guilt.

2.   **One who likes "interesting" cases.** At one new visit, I asked the doctor if she was willing to take on someone like me. She smiled and said yes. "I like patients like you. Keeps me thinking," she said, and I went home with a smile on my face. Even if she couldn't always answer my questions, I knew she was on my side.

3.   **One who will not imply you're faking it.** One doctor who put his arm around my shoulder and patted me instead of digging deeper, I never had enough respect for him to go back again.

4.   **One who listens to the whole story.** This is important. Doctors are busy, and they have a tendency (understandably so) to hear the first three symptoms and run with them. I've noticed this pattern because the majority of doctors I've seen have immediately wanted to check my thyroid based on the first things I mention. (See the chart in the next chapter on how to avoid this.)

5.   **One who understands having multiple conditions.** Doctors are so specialized now, a lot of us have several different doctors for our different conditions, all giving us different, and sometimes opposing, instructions. Though we have to have them, if possible it's great to have one general doctor who can help you stir all the stuff into one big conglomeration, like your body does.

6.   **One who is not stressful to visit.** I used to dread going to doctors. I hated how stupid I felt and how inept I became the moment I sat on that examining table. Doctors have a great power for good or bad, and our stress level when we go see them matters to our health.

Here are two wrong ways to see your relationship with your doctor:

1.   **You are the victim and your doctor is Superman.** If you expect him to solve all your problems in a single bound, this leaves you with no personal responsibility and blindly following everything the doctor says, then helpless disillusionment when he proves to be human and his office doesn't keep perfect track of everything.

2.   **You are the victim and your doctor is the enemy.** This perspective leaves you fearful of the medical world in general and avoiding treatment you may need, or angry and bitter against the "system," which is not healthy in any direction.

What is the right relationship to have with your doctor? In my opinion, the right way is to see yourself and your doctor/s as a team. The sickness is the enemy, and you work together to fight it. That means you carry some of the responsibility, but not the full weight of it. There's someone to go to with your research and theories and questions.

Just like dating, keep trying until you find the right one. A good doctor truly wants to help you as a person, and doesn't scowl when you walk into the room. He doesn't make you feel embarrassed if you ask questions or lecture you if you have side effects to a medicine he prescribed. You leave a good doctor's office with a sense that you're moving forward—you the team rather than you on your own.

After many years of feeling solitary or even rejected, medically speaking, being part of a team feels really, really good.

Therefore we do not lose heart. Even though our outward man is perishing, yet the inward man is being renewed day by day.

2 Corinthians 4:16

<u>Individual Or Group Study Questions</u>

1. Has your experience with doctor visits thus far been more positive or negative overall?

2. If negative, has your experience been influenced by thinking either:

   • You are the victim and the doctor is the hero?

   • You are the victim and the doctor is the enemy?

3. How would you rate the following in importance?

   A doctor who:

   • Listens without jumping ahead.
   • Believes you.
   • Is willing to try unconventional options.
   • Will keep searching for the core problem.
   • Is cheerful.
   • Is realistic.

   ACTIVITY: Insurance and your location can both limit your choices of doctors/specialists, but as far as your choices go, when looking for a new doctor/s, the internet is now a great place to read reviews by patients and potentially save yourself significant stress by avoiding doctors with low patient rating on the things that matter most to you.

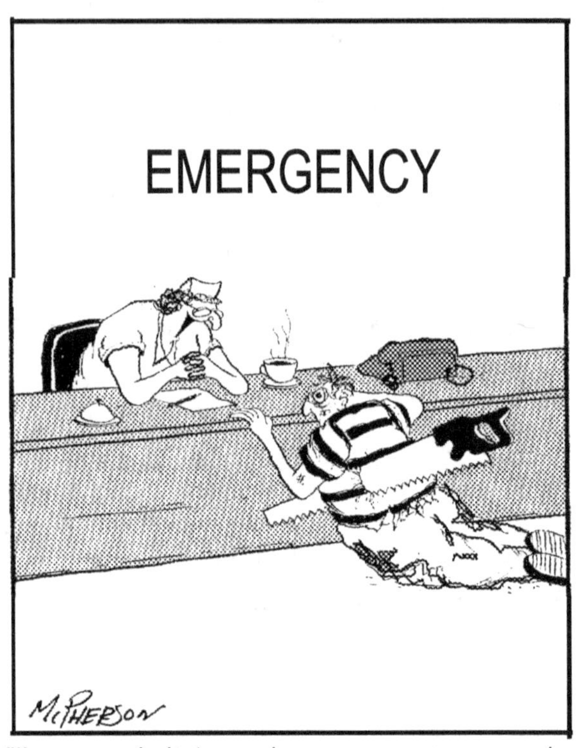

"I'm sorry, sir, but your insurance company requires that you first get a referral slip from your primary care physician before we can treat you."

Chapter Seven

Preparing For The Appointment

*Is there a medical rule that requires
doctors' office personnel to treat you
as though you have the IQ of a Cheeto?*

Dave Barry[ii]

You've decided to try a new doctor. You have an appointment scheduled, and your insides are already churning thinking about your typical pattern:

- Dread the appointment.
- Break out in a cold sweat once you step into the examination room.
- When the doctor walks in and asks how you are doing, you hear yourself say, "Fine."
- You start in on your long list of symptoms, but after three the doctor starts talking about what to test for.
- You end up nodding to whatever his idea is, thanking him, and leaving in a brain fog.
- Fifteen minutes down the road, you've thought of three questions you wanted to ask, one theory you had, and four more symptoms that the doctor should be aware of.

Don't you hate that? I used to look at doctor visits as for-sure failures. I never could seem to feel like anything more than a silent, helpless patient.

Over the past 20+ years, especially after I had my chart lost in a hospital and my name on somebody else's blood results (I'm so glad they caught that before treating me with whatever the other guy had!), I have learned to stop being so helpless and passive. I have become an involved and informed part-of-the-team patient, from the initial appointment, to treatment, to adjusting my medication, to getting answers to my questions even if the doctor is on her way out the door.

And in the hopes of sparing you a few years of misery, I'm going to share my strategy for going to a doctor's appointment. The following questions are for you to fill out before you go to the doctor, and from those answers you can create a sheet to take with you.

Actually you should create two sheets—one for the doctor and one for yourself with the personal stuff like your questions and your goals for the visit. I'm sure you already know that trying to keep it all in your head often doesn't work. There's something about doctor's offices that drains brain power, like going to the grocery store with five things in your mind, but the minute you see the hundred and seventy-two things on the shelf in front of you, those five things have run with wild abandon to some happy grocery-land oblivion where they can laugh at you from a distance.

Unofficial Questionnaire

for your upcoming Doctor's Appointment:

1.   **At what point did you know something was wrong?** What age? What symptoms?

2.   **Top/Worst three symptoms, then go lesser from there.**

3.   **What do you want from this appointment?** A prescription? Information? A diagnosis? What do you want the doctor to do for you?

4.   **What is the next step?** Who is responsible—you, doctor, office lady—to do the next thing in moving forward?

5.   **Your theories.** Things you think might be the cause/problem. Anything you would like to get tested.

6.   **Your questions.** What would you be upset to leave the office not knowing, i.e. does the doctor think he can help you? Is there any connection between symptom A and symptom B?

7.   **Previous health experiences.** What has already been tested? What were the results? What treatments have other doctors already tried?

I feel the need to mention to women that it would probably be beneficial to avoid listing anxiety/depression symptoms in your first three symptoms (unless those are your main problem, which would make them your main priority). Doctors see lots of women, particularly 20's to 40's who are tired, down, have no energy, are drained, anxious, irritable, etc. They have a standard treatment path they follow for that, so if you want to be considered outside that category, you need to present yourself outside that category so the doctor will not go to his default path in that direction.

Once you have filled out the above questionnaire, you will have a clearer idea of what you are hoping for from the visit, and what you can take into it to help the doctor help you.

I used to look at the doctor like he was some kind of magician who would examine me and check my heart and somehow know exactly what was wrong with me. I would actually get frustrated when he would keep asking me questions, assuming he should already know what my problem was.

Now I know that the doctor is going to try to help me, but I need to give him as much information as I can to help him do that. So I now have a history sheet. I also make sure I have in writing the questions I want answered, and check my list throughout the appointment to make sure each one gets covered. That way I leave feeling like my money and time were well spent, and I have a direction to go from there.

Two personal examples to show what I mean:

Back when I was looking at doctors with a little too much idealism, I went to one and tried to explain my symptoms, focusing on the one that disturbed me the most: this feeling of anger I would get that I didn't want and didn't understand. He left the room for a bit, then came back in with a set of papers. He patted me on the shoulder and told me I should consider that it might be depression, and from that moment I knew he was done. He had what he thought was my problem, so no need to look deeper. No tests. No bloodwork.

Now, to be transparent, I've been through a time of depression (there's a whole chapter on depression in *Why Doesn't God Fix It?*) and that wasn't it. I know now that was a clear symptom of my blood sugar dropping. In fact, even my real time of depression had major connections to physical problems that I didn't know I had at the time. The doctor was trying to be kind with the understanding smile and the patting, but I left that day feeling labeled and overlooked as a person and a patient.

Fast-forward about twenty years and seven diagnoses later. Now, having learned better how to present my problems, and also which buzz words to avoid, I went to my Endocrinologist to ask a very specific question. We went through the usual, checking on things regarding my adrenal problem and my daily dependent need for steroids. Then, when it was my turn to talk, I handed over my pain picture and asked my prepared question. With 30% to 50% of my body being in chronic pain due to Ehlers-Danlos Syndrome, what was I supposed to do? Pain is a stressor on the body, so just trying to endure the pain would not be good for my adrenal condition and cause me to need more steroids, which of course is not good. However, the only thing that dealt with the pain at that point was narcotics, and even they didn't fully take it away. You see, I knew narcotics were a big trigger topic, so just bringing them up would put me in a category. By addressing this with the two options, I showed that I wasn't taking them flippantly or because I was addicted, which is, for good reason, something they're worried about.

My doctor looked over my pain picture, which showed much more clearly than words that this was a genuine, daily problem. He looked me in the eye and said, "That's a tough one." We talked about how I was stuck in a difficult place, without a good option. I left that day with no miracle cure but with my self-respect intact.

To bring this all together, I'd recommend creating one sheet to actually hand over to your doctor, which helps him look at the big picture rather than processing a few symptoms and forgetting the rest. Having a sheet also puts his focus on facts on paper, a problem to solve, rather than listening while assessing non-verbals such as how you're dressed or nervous gestures that might send him in the wrong direction regarding whether or not you should be taken seriously. This sheet can be made from the answers to questions one and two. You could even try to impress him by putting the symptoms into categories like Gastrointestinal, Neurological, etc.

For yourself, create a sheet with the answers to questions three through six. If the doctor suggests a test you've already done, you've got all that information ready to give, rather than, "Well, I think a doctor checked that a few years ago and didn't find anything." This is blank information, meaning it tells him nothing so he has no reason not to do the test again. However, if you can tell him, "Doctor so-in-so at such-and-such place did an MRI three months ago. They didn't find any sign of a pituitary tumor. I have the report with me. Would you like to see it?" Boom, that's information that will help him.

When the appointment is winding down and the doctor asks if you have any questions, you aren't so full of his information that you don't remember what you wanted to say. You can check your sheet and bring up anything that wasn't covered.

This is a new habit that takes practice getting used to, but I have found it immensely helpful in making me feel part of the team working to find a solution. And it's nice to not be beating myself up all the way home from a fruitless visit because I suddenly remember what I went to the doctor for in the first place!

<u>Individual Or Group Study Questions</u>

Go ahead a get a head start on that questionnaire.

1. At what point did you know something was wrong?

What age?

What initial symptoms?

2. Write your top/worst three symptoms, then go lesser from there.

ACTIVITY: Type out a document of all you filled in above, then add the rest of the questions from page 49 below that. Save it on your computer so you have a template that you can use and adapt for different appointments. That way you don't have to start from scratch every time.

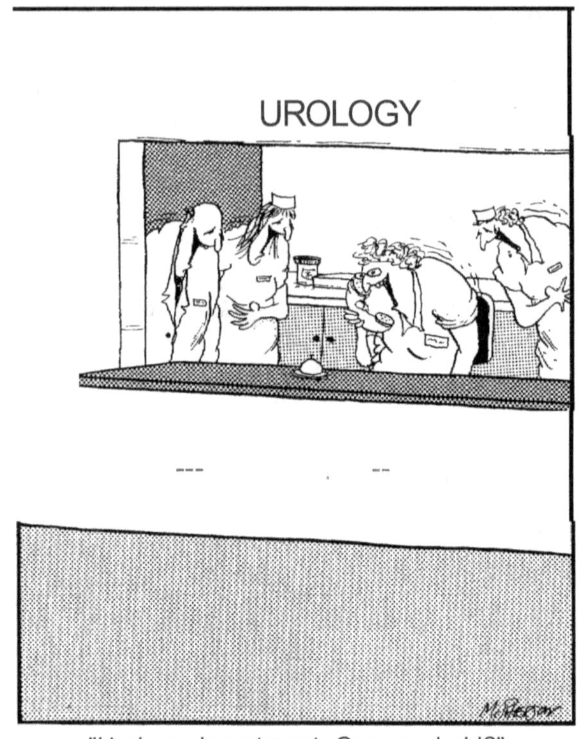

"Urology department. Can you hold?"

Chapter Eight

⌐◦⌐

Tests, Medication, And Side Effects

Half the modern drugs could well
be thrown out the window,
except that the birds might eat them.

Martin H. Fischer[iii]

My asthma had flared significantly enough and often enough that I needed help. I went to the asthma/allergy doctor yet again, and she sent me home with two new medications. One was prescription and one was a general nasal spray I could get over the counter. I bought the non-smelly version and was pleased at how much it helped. For me, taking something new and not having bad side effects is a plus, so I incorporated this new set of medications into my daily life and enjoyed the improvement.

Fast forward two weeks. You know how it is when you start feeling "off," but you can't quite tell if it's a genuine symptom or not? I was feeling that way, but of course that could always be due to lack of sleep or any number of other reasons. I wasn't trying any new medication, so dismissed that idea. As the days passed, however, that off feeling went dark. I started waking up at night with panic attacks. Fears and anxiety seemed to hover over me, with those awful adrenaline rushes that take over the whole body and don't subside for long, stressful stretches of time.

Real life is rarely as simple as a paragraph on paper. I know you have also experienced that difficult season of wondering if something is wrong, being sure something is wrong, not being able to pinpoint what it actually is, and then not being able to find the source once you do pinpoint it. It's a time of uncertainty and stress. For me, once I was sure this was not me and I was reacting to something, I started researching my medications, particularly those that were new to me.

I've discovered that checking standard medical sites tends to only give a sterilized version of information. If I want real information, I need to go to the people who have actually tried the medicine. I usually find them in forums online or asking questions online. There's no set way to find them. I have the most success putting a sentence in my search engine rather than a topic.

Example:

What will get standard medical results: Nasal Spray side effects.

What might get real people discussing the unusual stuff: I started using nasal spray two weeks ago... or I'm using nasal spray and having panic attacks at night...

I've found that typing in a sentence gets me more of the real-people questions and answers out there. Sometimes that can be very overwhelming, so it's not recommended unless you need information, but when needed, it has genuinely helped.

It took time, but I finally discovered that my innocent-looking, over-the-counter nasal spray had the long-term side effect of panic attacks. I stopped using it and the terrible symptoms went away.

My friend JD has also experienced long-term side effects that a doctor typically would not mention. She recommends we, "Make sure you check the side effects. This may sound like obvious advice but there is a curious delusion that happens. Two decades ago, I would hear, or read, side effects and think they wouldn't happen to me. Or, I would forget that new medications won't have the full list of side effects because not enough people have reported them yet. I have to admit I used to read the list of side effects and secretly think they didn't actually have side effects, those were just things they included to avoid being liable. If the side effects were true, why would they prescribe it? My doctors seemed to participate in this delusion and in some cases, actively denied side effects.

"I have also discovered that you have to keep checking because the doctor doesn't look at the list of symptoms you keep coming in for and check them against your medications and current, known side effects. I suffered incredible, increasing joint pain while on my first blood thinner. My doctors adamantly denied that the blood thinner had side effects other than excessive bleeding. The doctors kept trying to fix my symptoms by giving me anti-depressants because they had 'pain management' properties. A lot of doctors hear your symptoms and give you a pill. If the issue is a side effect of medication you're on, then taking more medications with side effects won't help you. I finally convinced a new doctor to switch my blood thinners and my joint pain decreased significantly.

"A decade later, after multiple trips to the doctor about my increasing dizzy spells, headaches and migraines, I discovered that they were reported side effects of the new blood thinner that were not reported when I started the new medication. Being aware of the side effects can also be important when considering changes in your body, health and mental state over time.

My neurologist gave me a medication to try and help with my migraines. It caused a huge emotional change. At one point I got so upset over something small I had the thought that I should just drive head on into traffic. I knew instantly that wasn't me and got home and called the doctor right away to tell him I wasn't taking those meds anymore. Some side effects take years to be noticeable. An occasional headache can turn into a daily occurrence, with weeklong migraines once or twice a month, through the course of years of silently enduring while no one can figure out what's wrong. It's so hard to stay hyper vigilant of your symptoms much less keep track of an ever-changing list of side effects, but it can be worth it. Being aware of the side effects means you can make choices about what side effects are, or are not, worth it to endure, and ultimately might reduce your medication list."

I totally agree, JD. I wish there was a way to make it easier on us than having to try things to see if the benefit is worth the side effects, but every body is different so what works for one person might be terrible for another. My sister appreciates a medication that, for me, caused bad emotional side effects. I think I might be taking the migraine medication JD mentioned and it helps me with pain, but she can't take it. We're all wired differently, and medication is made of chemicals that cause reactions. The intention is a good reaction, but we can't blithely assume if it's called medicine it will be good for us. That goes for holistic and supplemental options as well. Just because something is natural or organic doesn't make it good either, such as poison mushrooms or poison ivy.

Some people are afraid to try anything under the label of medication. Others feel the more the better. Again, a balance is to be desired. Medicine is a tool. The right tool can be wonderful. The wrong can be destructive. Too many tools gets confusing.

We need to remember that tools are created to assist us, not to overtake us. We are the experts on our own bodies. When you know something is wrong, take that seriously even if others don't.

I hope you are able to find a set of tools that will help you live well.

Be of good courage,
and He shall strengthen your heart,
all you who hope in the Lord.
Psalm 31:24

Individual Or Group Study Questions

1. Was is the strangest or scariest side effect of medication you have experienced?

2. Do you generally approach trying a new medication with:

   - Fear – I'm going to have every side effect on the list, plus a few more.

   - Optimism – This is definitely going to make things better.

   - Caution – It might help, it might cause problems, but it's worth the try.

   - Rejection – Medicine is chemicals and there has to be a holistic version that's just as effective.

3. Do you think medication is always good or always bad or it depends? How would you explain your answer?

ACTIVITY: If you have multiple new medications or supplements to try, create a plan of 2 weeks per new med, with the most important or potentially most helpful ones first. If the potential side effects are concerning, highlight the ones most important and have the paper someplace accessible so that, if need be, you can just pull out the paper and point if help is needed. This is very effective in Urgent Care – pointing at the paper gives them the medication and side effect and will save many steps and words of explanation.

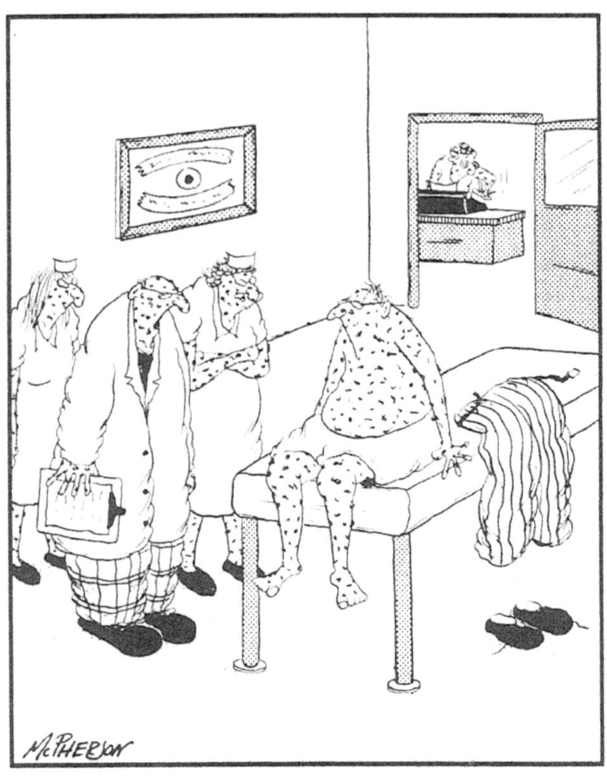

"We have no idea what you have, Mr. Schaad,
but whatever it is, it's extremely contagious."

Chapter Nine

When the Well-Meaning Annoy You

*I am at the moment deaf in the ears, hoarse in the throat,
red in the nose, green in the gills, damp in the eyes, twitchy in
the joints and fractious in temper from a most intolerable
and oppressive cold.*

Charles Dickens

I don't know about you, but sometimes I get tired of people trying to cheer me up. Not true friends who understand, but people with the pat answers. You know the kinds of things I'm talking about, things like:

"You can choose to be happy."

"Just believe God and you'll be fine."

"It's always darkest before dawn."

"It could be worse."

"_______________________________________"

I wish I could hear the ones you're saying right now. Go ahead and write them out. Write a whole page full if it'll make you feel better.

Regardless of whether the statements are true or not,

the problem is not the words but the tone, the facial expression, the underlying implication that if we'd just suck it up and smile, everything would be fine, and because we aren't, it's somehow our own fault.

It's like they think warm, fuzzy bugs are flying around, ready to settle upon anyone willing, so if we'd just read some *Chicken Soup for the Sickie-Head's Soul* (no, that edition hasn't come out yet), we'd welcome the warm fuzzies, be happy, and all our problems would go away.

Gag.

The truth is, there are some days I don't want to hear the right answers. I already know the right answers, but I'm so tired ... so very, very tired. And I'm tired of being tired. I'm tired of being so out of control, of not being dependable anymore. I'm tired of having to fight and fight every day in a war I know I can't ever fully win.

I want a break from having to constantly know what time it is so I don't miss eating exactly when I should. I want a day where I can eat anything I want, where I don't have to count carbs or sugar content or make sure I have enough protein. I want to not have to take pills at exactly the right time every single day.

I want a day off from being a sick person. I want to go back to being like the "normal" people around me, who take all those things for granted.

And I'm ashamed saying so. I know there are people far worse off than I am. I know I have so much to be thankful for.

And yet, there are certain times and certain days (and I'm annoyed and embarrassed saying it, but most often they have to do with my hormonal cycle—ugh) when it piles up, you know? I don't feel like focusing on sunshine and rainbows and lollipops. I can't eat lollipops anyway.

Those times, it's almost as if I'm tired of being strong and I just want to be miserable for a little bit. I feel yucky physically and I'm tired of the energy it takes to not feel emotionally yucky too.

Does this mean I'm a terrible person, or I don't have faith in God, or I need counseling?

I'm going to give you my theory on the yucky times. This isn't scriptural; it's just my opinion. Please check it out with God before you give it a green light.

The two most obvious options are to stuff the feelings or go with the feelings. Neither choice works out very well.

When I pretend I'm not feeling down and stuff it all, it builds up and erupts on someone, like my husband or kids, and then I feel even worse and more ashamed of myself, even more like a failure.

However, if I just excuse it and say I deserve to feel this way and let the feelings fly, I also end up crabbing out on others, or complaining, or some other action that dishonors God and doesn't make anyone around me happy.

So, is there some option that doesn't keep the feelings festering in me while also protecting all heads in the vicinity from being bitten off? I think there is.

It goes back to the accepting and adapting idea. First, I need to accept and admit I feel this way—to God, my husband, or a good friend. Just saying it out loud has healing properties in it. Then I need to adapt to the situation. In other words, if I can tell I'm up to my neck in frustration about my condition (not that it's worsened right then, just the fact of it, and the fact that it's not going away), I should change my situation so that others are not negatively affected by my feelings and the outward result of them.

In other words, I need to get away from people. Those are the times I ask my husband if he'd watch the kids so I can go away by myself and write. (This book may actually be more therapy for me than it is for you—don't take it personally.) I get away by myself and focus on something else, and somehow just a small break of a couple of hours can make a huge difference.

If you're not into writing, maybe it's something as simple as going into a room by yourself and watching a movie, reading a good book, or going shopping. (We'll talk more about that later in the series.) Giving yourself some kind of a break from the stress is a coping mechanism. It doesn't mean you can't handle your condition, or you're a failure. It means you're human and you sometimes get overwhelmed by a problem that never goes away. That sounds pretty normal to me.

In conclusion, if you catch yourself wanting to snap when someone offers you sunshiny thoughts or happy endings, it is my humble opinion that you should find a way to take a little break. Even a marathon runner needs to stop between races. Some of us don't get to take a break from our conditions for weeks, days, or even hours. But if you can find some way to forget about it or leave the responsibilities of it with someone else for a little chunk of time, I believe it will be good for you, for your family, and anyone else within head-biting range.

<u>Individual Or Group Study Questions</u>

1. What phrase do people say that gets to you the most?

2. Why? What do you feel it implies about you or your condition?

3. How do you want to respond? In your flesh? Be honest.

4. How do you usually respond (outwardly)?

5. Do you feel it's wrong to admit you are feeling frustrated with your condition? Why or why not?

6. What would feel like a break to you?

7. Who can help you get a break? Would they be willing?

ACTIVITY: Give yourself permission to take a break sometime this week. When you do, enjoy it without guilt.

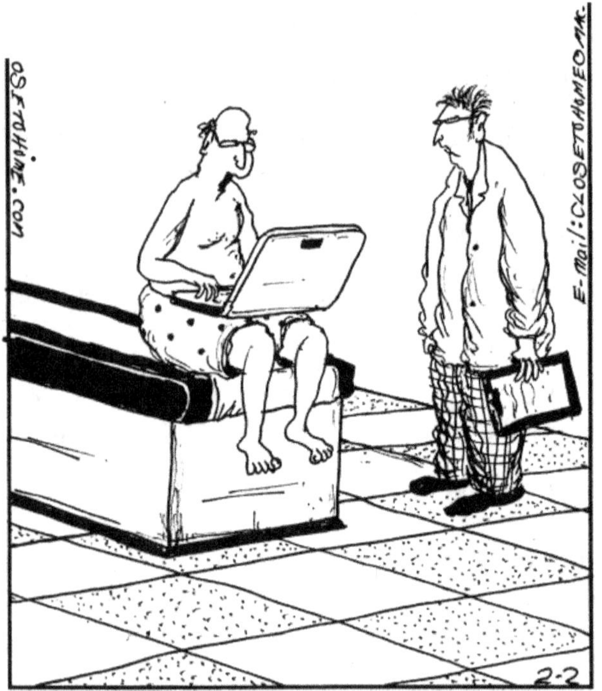

"Okee-dokey...let's just see how your diagnosis and treatmant plan compare to what Webmd.com has to say..."

Chapter Ten

But You Don't Look Sick!

Red meat is not bad for you. Now blue-green meat, that's bad for you!
Tommy Smothers

You know those little motorized sit-down cart thingies they have at Wal-Mart? I have needed to use them a time or two. I hated it, especially when I'd stand up out of the cart to reach something higher on the shelf. I was certain everyone was staring at me thinking, "Shame on her. She looks just fine. Why isn't she letting some little old lady use that thing? Or someone with a broken leg? She doesn't need it!"

I wanted to tell everybody I passed, "I know you can't see it, but I really am sick. Right now I would not have the strength to do my shopping if I had to walk through this big store. I'm sorry for using this resource when you don't think I should, but I really do need it."

Can you hear my subtle whimpering tone? Like a puppy that wants some attention but is scared you'll hit him?

Why do I feel the need to explain myself to random strangers who might or might not be judging me based on my outward appearance and their misconceptions of it? That's not reasonable.

But, oh so natural, right? We care about what people think of us. We don't want people whispering and gossiping behind our backs about how we must be faking it, or trying to get undeserved sympathy, or just wanting attention. Often we end up doing things that damage our health so people don't get the wrong impression.

Before you object and say you don't do that, look through the following:

Have you ever...

1. Stayed longer at an event than your body could handle because you didn't want people making conclusions about why you left early?

2. Kept from getting the food or rest or whatever your body needed because you were talking with people and did not want to express your needs, not wanting them to think that's all you ever talk about?

3. Told someone you were "just fine," when you really should have said you were struggling and needed prayer?

4. Put an extra layer of makeup on before church or work so people wouldn't know you'd been crying beforehand?

5. Walked through the store instead of using the motorized cart thingy because you felt others would think you weren't bad-off enough to deserve it?

6. Lifted things you shouldn't, kept from eating what you should, not taken your medication on time, etc. because you didn't want to show your condition to someone healthy you were visiting or talking with?

I doubt any of us could answer no to all these questions. Some of us have done every single one. We have all made the wrong choices at times because we care so much what people think of us.

No one likes being judged or misunderstood, which is why we want to defend ourselves when people say the very common phrase, "But you don't look sick!" Sometimes they say it out of bewilderment, sometimes out of a judgmental attitude, and sometimes they actually think they are being encouraging by letting us know we don't look like half-dead drowned rats, considering we are so sick.

I used to think it was my spiritual responsibility to make sure I never gave anyone reason to misunderstand or think incorrectly about me, my motives, or my actions. Was that ever exhausting! I was always second-guessing what I'd said or not said. I'd leave parties and spend hours worrying about the way people might have misinterpreted my comments. I would get tied up in knots before meeting with someone, already worried about what I was going to say wrong.

I was taking the verse about abstaining *from all appearance of evil* (1 Thessalonians 5:22) and translating it to mean, "Worry yourself sick over what everyone thinks about you because you're responsible to make sure no one ever thinks wrongly of you." That's not what it means. The more I studied the life of Jesus Christ, who was often misunderstood even though He was perfect, the more I noticed He did not chase people down trying to make sure they didn't get the wrong impression from His words or actions. In fact, He often said things that left people without the answers they were searching for and gave them more important questions to ponder.

There are always going to be people who don't understand. Always. We can make ourselves sick trying to prove our conditions to them—which isn't fun since we're sick already—or follow them around whimpering for their approval. We can even become angry and bitter over their lack of it.

Or we can leave them be, understanding this very important truth: We are not responsible to keep everyone from thinking the wrong thing.

If someone wants to be judgmental and think we're faking it or whatever, that is a problem between them and God, not them and us.

Did you get that? It's something between them and God, not them and you.

There are plenty of people who would like to understand, but their realm of experience just hasn't connected with chronic health issues yet. Few of us really understand anything other than what we ourselves have gone through, so even those of us within this group have trouble understanding those with conditions other than our own.

Many years ago, a friend was having a biopsy on her breast to check for cancer. I felt terrible for her and wanted to help. I waited for her at the hospital and when she returned, not knowing what to do or say (we weren't very close and she was shy, and shy people really intimidate me), I started asking questions about the procedure. I could see this made her uncomfortable, but I didn't know what else to do, so I kept talking.

Finally, she said plainly, "I'd rather not talk about this." That shut me up, in a good way. I was so relieved to finally know what she wanted, and that she wasn't expecting me to cheer her up or get her mind off it. We walked in silence, without me being all tied up in knots because I wasn't saying the right thing.

I had wanted to help, but didn't know what was needed.

This is important. I really think most of the time, when people do things that are insensitive or feel unkind, it's not that they don't care and are being malicious toward us. It's probably because they are uncomfortable and don't know what to do; therefore, they often do or say things unhelpful or even hurtful.

And this is *really* important—they can't change until they know what you want or need.

My friend Bethany, who tends to ignore or downplay her MS because she doesn't want people to think she's blaming God, was at church talking with people, not wanting to bring attention to herself by saying she needed to sit down, but her body was demanding it. Finally, she stated it, and not only did no one have a problem with her need, it actually turned out to be a blessing to an older woman who also felt better sitting down.

Had I been there, I would have loved to sit down with Bethany, but not knowing enough about her individual symptoms, I would not have guessed what she needed.

We've all judged others based on our wrong impressions. (See Ecclesiastes 7:21.) We shouldn't worry too much about others judging us. And truthfully, it's likely very few people are spending their time analyzing and assessing us and our motives. Most people are thinking of themselves, just like we are, worrying about what everybody is thinking about them.

So should we avoid taking the elevator to the second floor because people might think we're lazy? No. Take the elevator, and if you feel everybody glaring at you, try smiling and saying, "Sorry, I've got __________ and stairs really hurt." Wouldn't you feel more understanding if someone said that to you? And maybe that's what they'll think next time someone else takes the elevator to the second floor, or they'll become more compassionate in general. That's a great thing, isn't it? And you helped them get there.

Please don't apologize for what your body needs. Most people like to help, they just don't know what you need. And God blesses people when they help others, so you're actually providing opportunities for a blessing for them.

Therefore, for the nice people, tell them what you need already. The rest, don't bother taking on their issues. You have enough to deal with.

And if I see you in one of those Wal-Mart cart thingies, I'll try to smile at you, just to make you feel better. You do the same for me, okay?

<u>Individual Or Group Study Questions</u>

1. Do you feel a sense of guilt that your condition is not obvious enough to warrant everyone's belief?

2. Do you find yourself responding with:

   • Defensiveness, ready to argue?

   • A need to prove to everyone how bad it is?

   • Sensitivity—they shouldn't have said that?

   • Pity party—nobody understands?

   • Hiding and avoiding anyone who doesn't get it?

3. Again, do you think if you had a sense of confidence about your condition, it would transfer to those around you?

4. Do you think we are responsible for what people think of us? If so, to what extent?

5. How does not communicating what we need lead to misunderstanding?

   ACTIVITY: Find a loved one or friend who has a stable, solid personality. Ask that person if they will help you see clearly when you are struggling. If they are willing, those times when you are worried about what someone might think, call your friend, tell them the situation, then choose to believe them if they say that person's feelings are not your responsibility.

CLOSE TO HOME   JOHN MCPHERSON

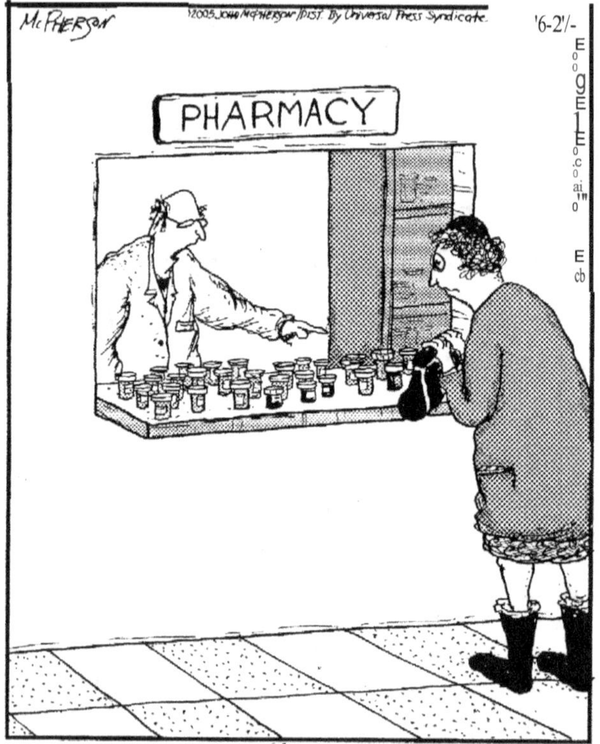

" ...which in turn will cause side effects of nausea for which I'm giving you Trylitol, which will induce temporary blindness, which I'll counteract with..."

Chapter Eleven

The High Cost of Going ... Anywhere

If you do everything you should do,
and do not do anything you should not do,
you will, according to the best available statistics,
live exactly eighteen hours longer
than you would otherwise.

Logain Clendening

When you have a chronic condition, it borders on amazing the amount of paraphernalia you have to take with you whenever you leave home, even on the smallest errands.

I have to take snacks in case I can't get to food exactly when I need it. I carry around an emergency shot/dose with needle in case—well, in case there's an emergency. I need my pills, whichever of my six prescriptions I'll need for the hours I'll be out. Then there's the sugar-free chocolate if I want to have something to eat while everyone else is eating dessert, the perfectly proportioned snacks for in-between meals, the carbonated, caffeine-free, sugar-free drink for when I have to ride in the backseat of a car since I get very motion sick, the sugar-free gum or mints in case I get nauseated, the medical bracelet I always have to wear, the glucose tablets in case I have a blood-sugar low, and of course, all the normal stuff people carry around, like a wallet and car keys.

And that's just for going out for a few hours. An overnight trip is even more fun.

For diabetics, it's a pain to carry around all the insulin they'll need, and to interrupt whatever event they're enjoying to go give themselves a shot.

For people with certain lung diseases, they have to be "beaten" every day, a ritual where someone has to hit them all around their back to break up the mucus, with their hand held in a cupping motion. This is definitely not something you can skip if you're at someone else's house, nor can you ask someone in line at the Post Office to do it for you since you're running late.

My mom has a funny little zapping machine for her back problems. She has to get it out at night and get all hooked up. It makes little beeping noises while it's doing whatever it does. If she's using it while a movie is playing, you start to think a bomb is getting ready to go off, which is pretty funny if you're watching an old black-and-white romantic comedy.

Oh, I forgot…I also carry around my inhaler. Being allergic to dust mites and mold, I can walk glibly into a store and if it has antiques, all of a sudden I find I'm having trouble breathing. I would make a great mold inspector. Invite me to your house and within thirty seconds I can tell you if you have a mold problem.

Other people have to pack humidifiers, oxygen tanks, heating pads, or wheelchairs. Some people have food allergies so unusual that going to a restaurant or a potluck becomes an extremely frustrating experience. Others, like me, can't get anywhere near a fun, marshmallow-roasting bonfire because of the smoke. That's kind of okay with me these days since I can't eat the marshmallows, but I do hate the attention I get trying to sneak out without making anyone feel badly that I have to leave, and without having to answer a bunch of questions about why I'm sneaking away like that.

It's annoying to do all you have to do to get out there into the world and be with people, and sometimes it doesn't feel worth the effort. This is especially true if you end up talking with someone who doesn't get your condition at all and makes those helpful comments like, "So you don't have a diagnosis yet?" with that tone that makes it clear they think you're making all of this up. Here you are trying to be as normal as possible with your condition, and they're implying you invented it to get attention.

You can smack mosquitoes that get under your skin like that, but not people, so sometimes we just want to give up and stay home and become hermits. But avoiding people and events is not healthy, and hey, we're already unhealthy, so we don't need to add anything more.

Part of the problem is risk. What if we have a flare-up at someone else's house? What if we commit to some event and end up falling apart right in front of everybody?

There's a movie from 1976 called *The Boy in the Plastic Bubble*. It's a fascinating story about a teenager who had no immune system, so they created a little sealed-in room where he lived. He could never go out, never experience anything, in order to stay protected.

In the end, the boy decided he would rather live life fully, despite the risk, than avoid the world just to stay safe. The movie ends with him riding off on a horse with a girl. I enjoyed the thought, but I was cringing inside, thinking about five minutes after the movie ended, when one germ caught up with that kid, what then?

What's my point? We have a choice to make on how much we will avoid in order to make life safer or easier for ourselves. It is definitely wise not to overdo it just to prove we're not really sick after all. We are sick, so it's silly trying to prove we aren't. However, we shouldn't decide to avoid everything simply because it's too much trouble, or it feels too risky.

Where is a good balance? That depends on you, your personality, and your condition. Besides normal things, like going to church and the grocery store, I have figured out I can plan about two or three people activities a week if I'm stable. More than that and my body starts wearing down, which leaves me vulnerable to sickness.

I went to my very first writing conference this past summer. I wasn't sure how it was going to go and, sure enough, my asthma flared up right when I got there, and my Addison's couldn't handle the major schedule planned for those three days. I ended up having to choose to go to only about half of the sessions, and even had to miss some of those to go back to the room and rest. There was too much walking and meeting new people and having fun—yes, even fun is problematic these days.

It was a great conference, but I don't think I'll be going again. I felt like it wasn't worth all the money and used-up health for only getting to attend a third of the program.

Other things are worth it, like giving up my nap sometimes because a friend drops by, or taking extra medicine so I can speak at a women's meeting.

We sick people can't live spontaneously, that's for sure. We have to plan ahead for a lifestyle that fits within our limitations, and then prepare fully to have all the stuff we need to live that life, complete with a few just-in-case additions.

If you're just getting started into this unhealthy thing, be encouraged. It does get easier. As you go, you learn what is too much for your body to handle. You learn which activities—and which people—are exhausting, and which are invigorating. In time, it becomes a habit to put on the medical bracelet or count out the pills you'll need or grab an extra snack for the road.

Life is about more than being sick; we just have to bring a few extra things into that life ... just in case.

Individual Or Group Study Questions

1. Do you get frustrated at the lack of spontaneity in your life now that you have a chronic illness?

2. Which settings are most difficult for you?

3. Are there fun settings where you can enjoy yourself despite your illness?

4. Can you shift your schedule to do less of the difficult and more of the fun?

   ACTIVITY: Write a list of what you need to bring for certain activities. If you have different needs for different types of activities, write one list for each. Keep the lists available so you don't have to think through what you need every time an activity comes up.

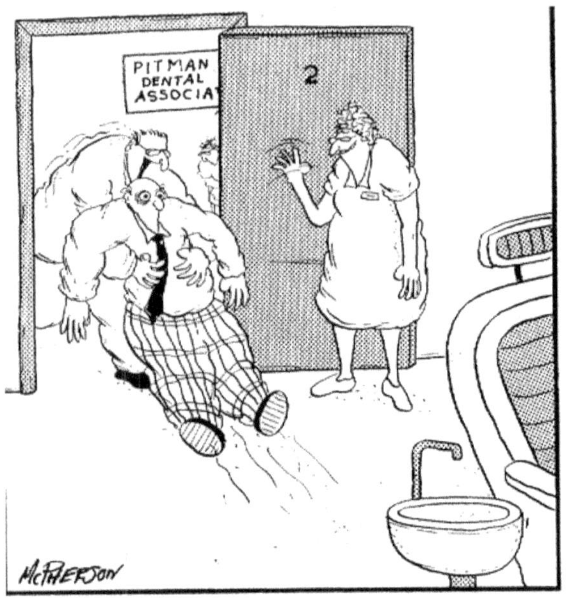

"You're just more affected by Novocain than most people, Mr. Cromley. You should regain full use of your legs in a day or two."

Chapter Twelve

Who Am I Now?

There are more pleasant things to do than beat up people.
Muhammad Ali (on one of his retirements)

I was twenty-two years old when I traveled to Bangladesh, one of the most colorful, chaotic, exciting places in the world. The day I arrived, the second largest Muslim festival in the world was letting out right around the airport and what should have been a fifteen-minute ride to the guest house took over three hours of jostling, honking, and edging forward inch-by-inch while millions flowed around us in brightly painted baby taxis, rickshaws, and even on foot.

Bangladesh is extremely crowded. Being out in the city felt like shopping on the day before Christmas. I thrived on all that adventure and noise and color and life.

In the ensuing years, I rafted the Nile River in Uganda, got to see Mt. Everest on a trip to Nepal, and ate cow brains just to say I'd done it. I went to amazing places, tried amazing food, and met amazing people.

Fast-forward a few years. I am now thirty-seven and feel about sixty-five. Well, maybe older since I have seventy-year-old friends who can run circles around me. I now like quiet hours out in nature. I sometimes stay home from events because all the meeting and greeting is too exhausting, and I avoid chaos and crowds whenever I can.

Who am I? What happened that changed me from one type of person to another? How is it possible that health problems could not only change my body so much, but my personality and preferences too?

And which one am I really? The person I was before health problems, or the person I am now?

I'm both, which is really strange. I still remember the old me, the one who loved adventure and excitement and had big plans for traveling the world and rescuing orphans and making an impact. She was vivacious and energetic.

Over the past years, that part of me has deflated like a balloon. Even my mind has changed, because what used to be fun now has such unpleasant ramifications, those things don't appeal to me anymore. Like roller coasters. I used to love amusement parks and intense rides and now just the thought makes me nauseated. See, I do sound like an old lady already. (No offense to old ladies.)

Technically speaking, having Addison's means my body doesn't have the cortisol it needs to handle stress. That includes the things we naturally think of as stress, like injury, sickness, or conflict, along with the daily stresses of driving in traffic, balancing the budget, or even something as simple as a change in the weather.

For a while I wondered if I was making more out of this than was really legitimate—like overcompensating or being a hypochondriac.

Then I read about a study on rats. They took the adrenal glands out of these rats and as long as every single thing in their lives stayed exactly the same, the rats were fine. However, when anything changed—the temperature, food, schedule, anything—they dropped dead.

Wow, that's some serious validation.

Whether you are newly ill or have battled chronic illness for years, you probably struggle with the fact that not only has your body changed, you yourself have had to change because of it.

People who were big into athletics have to become couch potatoes (which is a way to stay big but not athletic). People who used to love cooking now hate it because they can only eat gluten-free. People who used to be exceptionally tolerant now find themselves irritated regularly, at others and even themselves.

And some of us, who used to enjoy living on the edge, now start backing away anytime we hear a kid in the store coughing, and we see ourselves getting out our anti-bacterial hand soap even though we used to get annoyed at people who did that sort of thing.

What has happened? Who have we become? And can we ever learn to like this new person?

I don't have a lot of big answers for that. In truth, I don't have any answers for that.

But one thing I do know is this: Even though I change, God does not. My identity is not in who I was or who I am, but in who God declares me to be. And when He declared me worth dying for, He did that knowing every stage of me—the healthy and the unhealthy. My worth to Him has not changed.

You may be feeling a little lost right now. You don't understand what is happening to your body, to your life, to your identity. You're starting not to recognize the person in the mirror anymore. Where do you put the person you used to be, and how do you make room for this person you have become?

Well, for one, don't freak out. I know that's not deeply philosophical advice, but it's easy to fall into the I-can't-help-it syndrome and let these new struggles take over. We used to never struggle with fear, now we're biting our fingernails to the quick. We used to never avoid sick people, now someone with the hiccups makes us nervous. It's easy to start saying we can't help being nervous, or angry, or irritable, or afraid.

We have been ushered into a new world where so many things are unfamiliar. And change is scary. But even if everything changes, God has not changed, and He will equip this new you just as He equipped and helped the you that you used to be.

This series of books is here to help too. All your questions won't be answered, because you probably have some questions only God knows the answer to. I can't help with those, not being God, but I can let you know you're not alone. What you're feeling is not abnormal, and there is hope, even in this new and frightening unhealthy world you now live in.

You may not really know who you are some days, but it's okay, because God does, and He loves you—both of you.

Individual Or Group Study Questions

1. What has had to change about you because of your illness?

2. Do you feel like a stranger to yourself because of the changes that have come from having an illness?

3. What do you miss about who you used to be or what you used to be able to do?

4. Before, when you were healthy, did you ever dedicate yourself—your life and your body—to God, for whatever purpose He had for you?

5. Do you believe God could have a purpose for your life still, even in your illness?

   ACTIVITY: Either alone or before witnesses, dedicate your life—the life you have now, who you are right now—to God for whatever His purpose is. Verbally accept that God has allowed even this illness in your life, so He will work it for good.

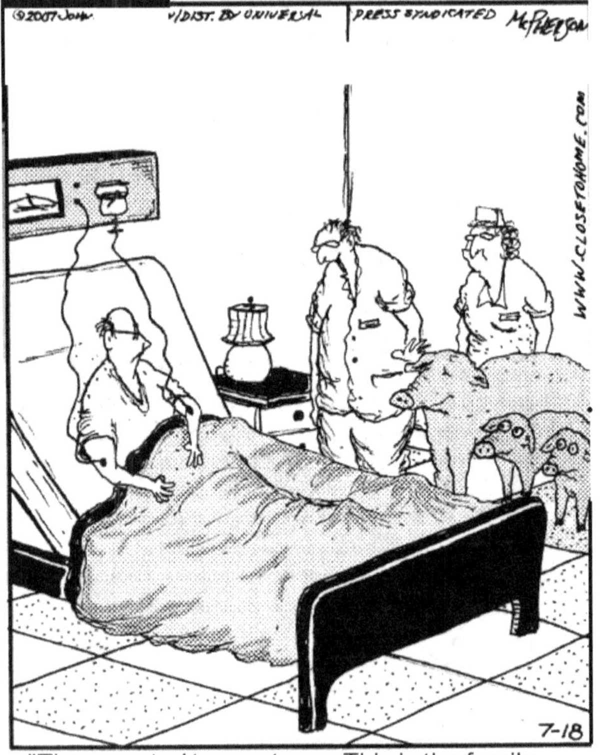

"They wanted to meet you. This is the family of 'Mongo,' the pig who donated the valve to you."

Chapter Thirteen

The Belief Test

Perhaps instead of asking questions of our trials;
our trials are meant to ask questions of us.

Esther, One Night with the King

Not long ago, I had to have an MRI to see if I had a pituitary tumor which might be causing my adrenal problems. The results came back that my pituitary was fine...meaning the adrenal problem is not caused by a foreign entity...meaning I have a lifelong incurable disease.

The MRI did, however, expose a cyst—or possibly a tumor—in a different place in my head. Not exactly what I had been hoping to hear. In the weeks between getting that news and talking to a top neurosurgeon at Emory about what to do about it, I struggled back and forth with my feelings like an emotional schizophrenic.

How did it feel to find out I have a cyst deep in my brain? In a physical sense, I felt no different. The cyst has likely been there for years. The symptoms did not change just because of this new knowledge of their source. But news like this brought out feelings that extended beyond the physical. I floated, dazed, from feeling this could not be really happening, to peace at God's higher plan, to a glimmer of hope that maybe fixing this could fix multiple issues, to the sobering knowledge that, *"The surgical removal of pineal region tumors ranks among the most difficult neurosurgical operations,"*[xiii] said one website.

Spiritually, I wondered what it all meant, while also knowing it was for God to know and for me to trust. Perhaps His purpose was to use this in some great way. Or perhaps the greatest purpose was for me to nestle closer to Him than ever before, knowing the peace that passes all understanding.

This latest health crisis was a gift, wrapped up in a test. Not a test by a hard taskmaster who wanted me to fail, but a loving Teacher, who wanted to show me not only where I am strong, but where I am weak; and in that weakness, to show His perfect strength.

Here are four things I believe:

1. God is good.

2. God loves me.

3. God could eliminate this problem at any moment and, therefore, because He has not, He has a reason.

4. God will do what is best.

My new circumstance did not make God any less good, or His love for me any less perfect. The question was, did I really believe what I say I believe? And herein is the test. Do I only believe God is good when He is doing what feels good to me? Or do I believe He is good no matter what? This is why tests and trials are gifts. They take us past the truths weighted down by our own understanding and into the place of truth that is eternal.

Here's why I think chronic physical difficulties can be gifts from God:

1. They remind us our lives and our bodies are not really our own.

2. They remind us not to take life for granted. We're not guaranteed tomorrow.

3. They keep us humble, as we have to ask for help and support from others.

4. They remind us of our need for God's daily help and presence.

5. They remind us every breath, every beat of the heart, every part of the body that is working, is a constant gift from God.

6. They teach us to accept that we can't fix everything, and that's okay.

7. They force us to have courage, to face our fears, to accept what we cannot change, because if we could, we would.

8. They force us to prioritize what matters most, because we physically cannot maintain lives filled with extra things.

I finally got to talk with the neurosurgeon, but I did not get the answer I wanted. Now, as I face this latest trial, I long to do so courageously, with joy and my face to the sun. Past the feelings and the flesh that want to give in to fear, anxiety and the doubt of unanswered questions, into the place of true peace, the place that knows my God is doing what is right. *For God has not given us the spirit of fear, but of power and of love and of a sound mind* (2 Timothy 1:7).

Individual Or Group Study Questions

1. What has been your biggest disappointment regarding your illness so far?

2. Do you feel like this illness is (mark as many as you feel are true):

   - Your own fault? If I'd only...

   - Someone else's fault? Doctor, negligent family, etc.

   - God's fault? If He really loved me...

   - God is punishing you for something?

   - God has forgotten about you or doesn't care about you?

   - God didn't give this, but He has allowed it for some reason?

   - God wants to use it for something good?

3. Do you believe God is good and He loves you? Why or why not?

4. Do you believe God could take away your condition if He wanted to, so since He hasn't there must be a reason?

5. Do you feel it's unfair for you not to be informed of what that reason is?

   ACTIVITY: Read through the eight reasons the author thinks chronic physical difficulties can be gifts from God. Highlight the ones you agree with. Underline the ones you don't. Then show the page to a friend, or God, and ask what they think about the underlined ones. Could there be truth you are missing

Conclusion

What Next?

If I had my way I'd make health catching instead of disease.
Robert Ingersoll

So where are you in all of this? Just found out you have a chronic condition? Had one for years? Somewhere in between?

Wherever you are on this health-issue journey, I welcome you to the Unhealthy Club with much sympathy, but also with a word of encouragement. You can do this. You'll have good days and you'll have bad days. You will struggle with accepting this, and even after you think you have accepted it, you will still sometimes find yourself struggling again.

That's okay. One very important thing to remember in all of this is that you are human. The Bible says God knows we are *but dust* (Psalm 103:14). We sometimes, however, seem to think of ourselves as failed superheroes who should be leaping tall buildings with a single bound—if only we could work up the energy.

If God remembers we're just well-arranged dirt and

creates His expectations of us accordingly, perhaps we could do the same, for ourselves and for others.

Here's my big final advice for this first book in the *Sick and Tired* series. Give some grace to yourself (let yourself be sick, admit it to others, ask for help), and give some grace to others (let your loved ones grieve as well, or get frustrated sometimes). All the gaps created by your illness...let God fill them up however He sees fit.

This life is a beautiful adventure, even if we can't run as fast as most of the people around us, and some of us can't run at all. Let's stop thinking of ourselves as chronic- health-problem-people and start thinking of ourselves as people who have chronic health problems. There is a difference. The difference is, you are more than your health problems.

God sees that about you. So do I. Now go look in a mirror and tell yourself:

You matter.

You are valuable.

Having a health problem has not changed that at all. You are not alone.

Till the next installment, walk with God, rest in God, and keep hope.

APPENDIX: Practical Pages

With all these tips and nuggets of advice, don't feel pressured to try everything, or anything. Think of this book as an information store. You can browse around, pick up a few, take one or two home, and return what doesn't work. Happy shopping!

Before the Appointment – my personal stash:

List of medications – pre-typed so I don't have to think through it every time.

List of symptoms – avoiding fatigue or anxiety if possible so I'll be taken more seriously.

Pain drawing – drawing of stick person with circled sections where I'm in pain, and maybe even arrows with other symptoms.

Something to do in the waiting room that is calming – funny book, work-type stuff to keep my mind off it, Kindle. Or I think through what I'm going to say and how I'm going to say it, prepping myself like an interview because in a way it is.

During the appointment:

When the doctor comes in and asks, "How are you today?" I've learned to say something like, "I need your help." This is a good statement because:

1. It shows I've got a need.

2. It implies I believe the doctor can help, which makes him feel more positive about this appointment.

3. It makes me sound legitimate – I've got an issue, but I'm not a hypochondriac, and I will be a reasonable person to talk with.

After the appointment I try to let myself have a de-stressor, like getting a specialty decaf coffee, or going for a walk to get out all that pent up angst.

After the Appointment - new medications:

1. When possible, don't try more than one new thing at a time, so you know what's causing any new side effects.
2. Have a specific place in your house for your meds and specific times you take them.
3. Create a way to show if you've taken them for the day already, such as laying them on the side if you took them, then at night putting them all back upright again. Or use those nice little compartment containers where you can set out a whole week's worth at once.
4. When taking something new, keep the side-effect sheet handy. You may want to show potential side effects to a family member or caregiver. If you start experiencing bad ones, you can simply point to the paper and they'll understand this is due to the medication and they need to get you help. (Once I took a paper to Urgent Care with the "potentially fatal" side effects highlighted that I was experiencing. They got me back to see the doctor quickly that day!)

<u>**Tips for testing:**</u>

Blood Draws:
1. Drink lots of water beforehand.
2. If you're a bad stick, or have a good arm, say so.
3. If you hate getting "stuck," use your good hand to pinch yourself somewhere else and focus on that.

Queasiness:
1. Peppermint to suck on or peppermint oil to smell.
2. Wet washcloth on the back of the neck.
3. Saltine crackers if you can eat.
4. Carbonated drinks can help.

MRI:
1. If you're claustrophobic, lay down, put a washcloth over your eyes, and don't look at the size of the testing hole as you're wheeled in. The washcloth will keep you from being able to sense the closure above you, and if you don't know how small or big it is, you're less likely to panic.
2. Quote Bible verses or pray during the test. Tell yourself they are doing their job and you don't need to think about the test at all. Put your thoughts on something else.
3. If you're struggling, focus on the "panic button" in your hand, and tell yourself you can push it in ten seconds. Count to ten. Then if you can, decide you can make it ten more seconds.

SICK & TIRED SERIES SPECIAL ADDITION

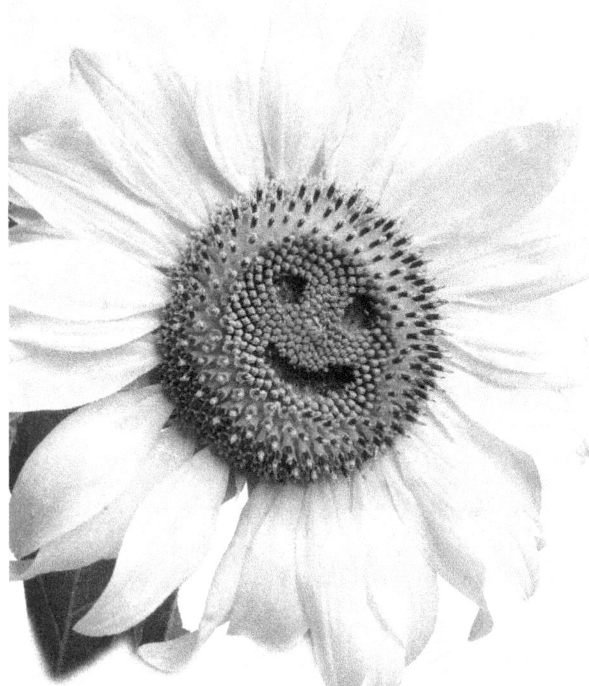

LAUGHTER
FOR THE SICK & TIRED

For The Days You Are Close To Crying and Wish You Had Something To Laugh About Instead!

Kimberly Rae

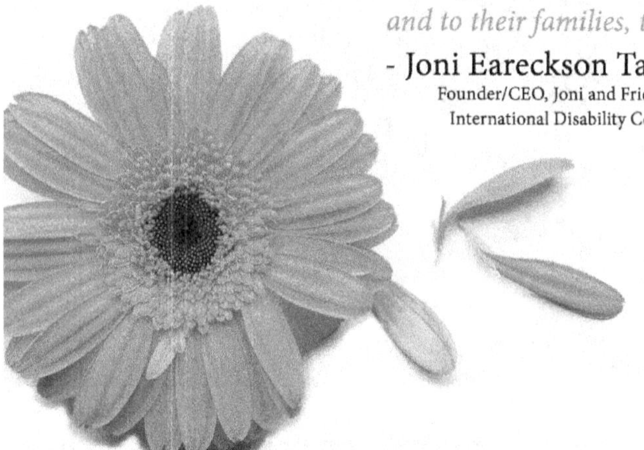

WHY DOESN'T GOD FIX IT?

Shining Eternal Light on the Darkness of Chronic Illness and Any Suffering

Kimberly Rae

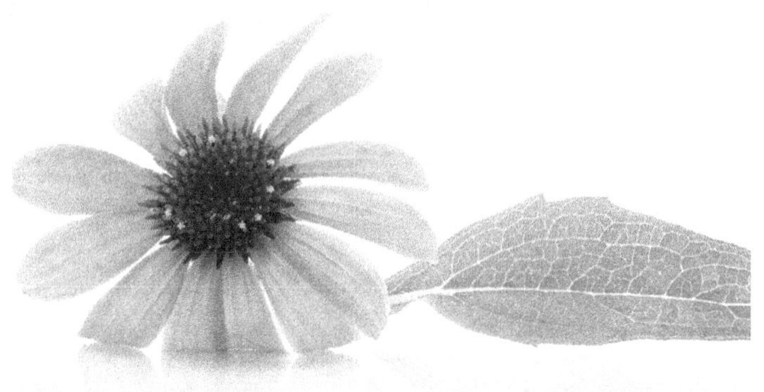

HELP FOR THE SICK & TIRED

Advice, Encouragement and Humor
From Those Who Understand

Kimberly Rae

*I have loved you
with an everlasting love.*
– God, Jeremiah 31:3

ABOUT THE AUTHOR

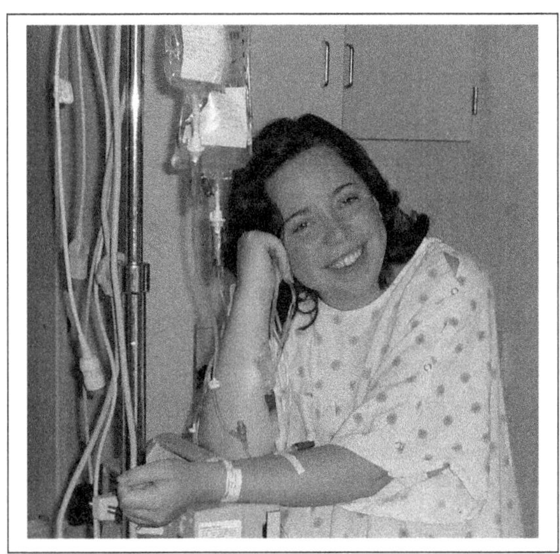

Kimberly Rae has been published over 200 times and has work in 5 languages. Future books in her Sick & Tired series follow along as Kimberly is diagnosed with Ehlers-Danlos syndrome and Chiari Malformation, a brain defect that really does make it all in her head. Rae had brain surgery in 2017, which made a lot of things much better and a few things worse.

Rae currently lives in Madison, Georgia, with her husband and two teenage kids.

Find out more at www.kimberlyrae.com.

Endnotes/Bibliography

http://www.brainyquote.com/quotes/quotes/m/marktwain105716.html

http://www.wired.com/culture/culturereviews/magazine/17-04/st_best

http://www.quotationspage.com/quotes/Robert_Orben/

http://www.quotationspage.com/quote/3238.html

http://www.cdc.gov/chronicdisease/overview/index.htm

http://www.restministries.org/media/statistics.htm

http://www.1-funny-quotes.com/funny-health-quotes.html

http://www.brainyquote.com/quotes/keywords/penguin.html

http://www.quotegarden.com/health.html

http://www.quotegarden.com/health.html

http://thinkexist.com/quotes/logain_clendening/

http://www.inspirational-quotes-cafe.com/inspirational-retirement-quote.html

http://neurosurgery.ucla.edu/body.cfm?id=1123&ref=77&action=detail

http://www.quotegarden.com/health.html

[i] https://www.brainyquote.com/topics/medical

[ii] https://www.funny-jokes-quotes-sayings.com/hilarious-short-quotes.html

[iii] https://www.brainyquote.com/quotes/martin_h_fischer_105721